A Study of
Buddhist Medicine and Surgery in Gandhara

INDIAN MEDICAL TRADITION SERIES

General Editors
DOMINIK WUJASTYK
KENNETH G. ZYSK

Vol. XI

A Study of
Buddhist Medicine and Surgery in Gandhara

DR. NASIM H. NAQVI

MOTILAL BANARSIDASS PUBLISHERS
PRIVATE LIMITED • DELHI

First Edition: Delhi, 2011

ISBN : 978-81-208-3502-3

MOTILAL BANARSIDASS
41 U.A. Bungalow Road, Jawahar Nagar, Delhi 110 007
8 Mahalaxmi Chamber, 22 Bhulabhai Desai Road, Mumbai 400 026
203 Royapettah High Road, Mylapore, Chennai 600 004
236, 9th Main III Block, Jayanagar, Bangalore 560 011
Sanas Plaza, 1302 Baji Rao Road, Pune 411 002
8 Camac Street, Kolkata 700 017
Ashok Rajpath, Patna 800 004
Chowk, Varanasi 221 001

Printed in India

By Jainendra Prakash Jain at Shri Jainendra Press,
A-45, Naraina Phase-I, New Delhi 110 028
and Published by Narendra Prakash Jain for
Motilal Banarsidass Publishers Private Limited,
Bungalow Road, Delhi 110 007

To my parents who gave me the
gift of education in the face
of most testing times.

Contents

Foreword

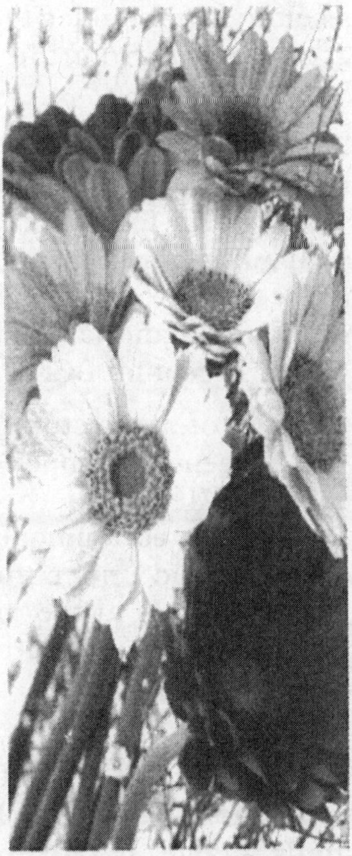

Gandhara was an ancient kingdom in the far north-west of South Asia, occupying the region that today lies across the borders of eastern Afghanistan and northern Pakistan. Its principal cultural centres were the cities of Puṣkalāvatī, Puruṣapura and Takṣaśilā (modern Charsada, Peshawar and Taxila). The kingdom of Gandhara lasted from the early first millennium BCE to the early eleventh century CE, but was at its cultural peak under the Kuṣāna dynasty of Buddhist kings who ruled from the first to the fifth centuries CE.

Gandhara was connected to the rest of the subcontinent by the famous ancient Northern Trunk Road (Sanskrit *uttarapatha)*, which formed a southern spur of the Silk Route. It was connected to the eastern Mediterranean by the trade route through the Parthian kingdom from Antioch to Kandhar that is described in Greek sources of the first century BCE.

At an early period of its history, Gandhara was politically part of the Achaemenid empire of Persia. Later, Taxila was captured by Alexander the Great, and his successors in the region created a unique blend of Greek and Asian art. After a period under the control of the Mauryan dynasty, Gandhara was in the third century BCE once again controlled and influenced by Greek culture through the Graeco-Bactrian rulers.

It has long been known that several ancient authors of ayurvedic treatises were residents of this complex, multicultural, vibrant region. The author Puṣkalāvata, from the city of the similar name, is said to have written a treatise on surgery, now lost. The Gandharan physician

Nagnajit, sometimes thought to be of a royal line himself, is remembered as an expert in toxicology. The famous physician Jīvaka, known from Buddhist sources, is said to have studied medicine at the university in Taxila, where some sources name his teacher Ātreya, describing him as a surgeon. The Ātreya Punarvasu, who taught medicine to Caraka and other founders of ayurveda, was probably different from Jīvaka's teacher, but nevertheless is also sometimes described as teaching medicine in Gandhara on one occasion. Some ancient legends place Caraka himself at the court of the Gandharan king Kaniṣka.

It has long been recognised that one of the wonders of ancient Indian medicine was its sophistication and innovation in the field of surgery. A wide range of specialized surgical instruments is described in such detail in the Sanskrit texts that it has been possible for modern museums to create accurate reproductions of them for display. Until now, however, no original instruments have been known to have survived from antiquity. Dr Naqvi's re-examination of the archaeological evidence from Gandhara, however, has now changed the picture, for it seems that we do indeed have ancient instruments that were simply not recognised as such by earlier generations of archaeological interpreters. Dr Naqvi offers a new interpretation of the archaeological evidence from Gandhara that sheds important new light on the history of ancient Indian surgery.

In short, Gandhara appears to have had a unique role in the medical history of South and Central Asia, and specifically the earliest history of surgery. This role was not unconnected with the Buddhist culture of the region. But until now, no special study has been dedicated to this topic. We are therefore happy indeed to present Dr Naqvi's new monograph in the series *Indian Medical Tradition.*

Dominik Wujastyk
Kenneth G. Zysk
January 2011

Figures and Illustrations

Preface

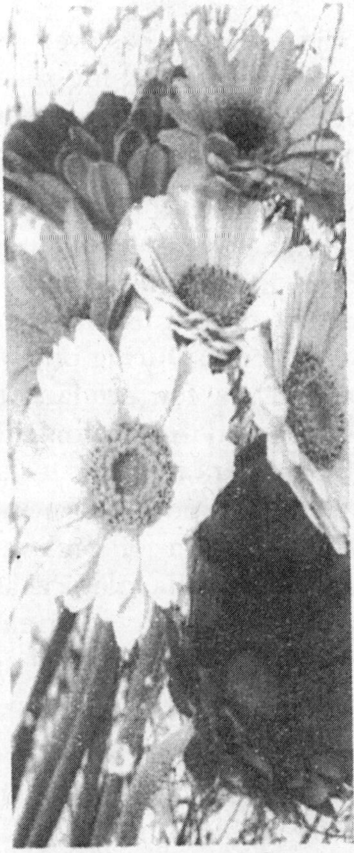

Why must I write this book? This question deserves a convincing answer and I had at least convinced myself before starting or even think about the title of the book. There are three good reasons why I wanted to put the facts on paper in respect of the study I had carried out regarding the practice of medicine and surgery by the Buddhists of Gandhara.

Firstly, it is a subject no one has ever treated before; an obvious fact when one starts searching relevant data in the literature of history of medicine regarding the medical achievements of the Buddhists in Gandhara.

Secondly, because I did my schooling in the neighbourhood of Taxila I always wanted to find more about its past and the social life of the people who built those monasteries, sculpted that art and made the objects that I saw displayed in the museum. During one of the many visits to the Taxila Museum I saw few artefacts that looked like surgical instruments. This led to a prolonged study of history and archaeology of Gandhara in order to understand these objects and culminated in a publication in *Medical History*. From this I always wanted to tell a comprehensive background story collaborating fully the archaeological assessment of the surgical and medical artefacts unearthed by the archaeologists in the light of their expert appraisal.

Thirdly, being an anaesthetist (anaesthesiologist) for 40 odd years and watching surgical procedures closely I had observed the improvements in the outcome within my practicing life were so visible, which I always attributed to unremitting advance and improvements of the available tools, a process that can be traced to the time of Celsus or even before. The evolutionary enhancements in instrumentation helped to improve the skills of both the surgeons and anaesthetists. A new blood pressure monitor or a modified surgical clamp, a hip implant made from a better metal or an inert plastic intraocular lens, all such new innovations consistently produced much better results than the previous versions. The opportunity of working in operating theatres, anaesthesia and intensive care surrounded by today's rapidly changing technology was a great help and inspiration. The fascination for instrumentation made me an avid collector of medical antiques and induced a passionate interest in the evolution of surgical instruments. My curiosity in the surgical instruments discovered from the sites of Gandhara was natural upshot from my hobby.

The excavated objects are silent witnesses, though they cannot speak but can make credible eyewitness if suitably analysed. The method employed in the study is comparison with known instruments from Greek and Roman period. Such an approach is reflected in the selection of the pictures where an effort is made to highlight by comparison the fact that in general design, size, shape and function most of the instruments, equipment and pharmaceutical related objects excavated in Gandhara do bear a resemblance with the acknowledged Roman or Greek objects despite the fact that their design was independently evolved by the people living far away from each other. Such a comparative study is intended to bring about an interesting emphasis for the reader who can see the essential details in two different objects at a glance and then makes an unbiased opinion regarding the argument. In search of surgical instruments of the period I have visited most museums in Pakistan, the National Museum at Delhi and in order to look at the real Roman and Greek surgical instruments I have also travelled to the National Archaeological Museum at Naples and the Museum at Epidaurus in Greece. While relevant information from some other such as Museum of Calcutta, Madras Museum (still known by old names), and Allahabad Museum was obtained by correspondence.

The consequence of the study of the surgical tools evidently ricochet on to the social history of the blacksmiths who made them, doctors or surgeons who used them and the patients who might have benefited or suffered from them.

These are the reasons why I wanted to write this account in a book form and I hope the readers may agree that at least I have tried to put most if not all relevant interesting facts together. This may not be a complete story but I have made a start to which more would surely be added by others in future. The process of finding the truth will continue.

Now by assessing the contents of the book it is also up to the readers to judge whether the question that was posed in the first line has been justifiably answered.

I would also like to bring to the notice of the readers two aspects at this stage. The spellings of Arabic, Sanskrit and Chinese names and words are not standardised and various texts have used dissimilar spellings causing confusion and even difficulty for their readers. Here a simplified version of the spellings is chosen from previous publications and applied throughout the text, with the hope that the choice will be undemanding and the readers will not be burdened needlessly. The readers may find at times repetition of events, if an account is echoed it was only to keep the subject matter in the context.

Finally I would like to take the opportunity to thank the Directorate of the Archaeology and Museums Government of Pakistan for granting me permission to photograph the exhibits and the staff of Taxila Museum for the help they provided during the photography. Thanks are also due to Mr. Saleh Muhammad Khan, the curator of the Peshawar Museum who was kind enough to allow me to photograph the Kanishka's Casket at the Peshawar Museum.

Introduction

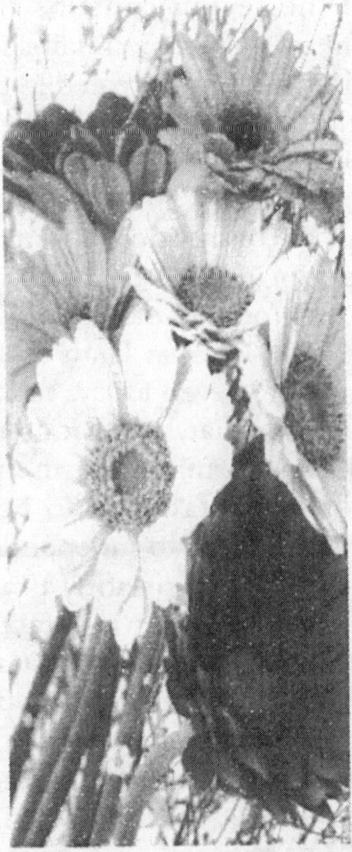

During the ancient times the territory of the present northern area of Pakistan and adjoining regions such as Afghanistan, part of eastern Turkistan was known as Gandhara. It is also a fact of history that never at any point in the past any borders were recognised to make Gandhara as a well defined state with recognised borders. Even though the geography of the region contains the most natural borders in the form of highest mountains in the World and the great rivers; this should have created lasting geographical boundaries. But the area always remained and still is the most porous, its inhabitants have always moved freely without any restrictions. From second millennium BCE till present this rugged region on both sides of some of the highest mountains in the World and their snow covered peaks remained a melting pot where a number of diverse civilisations arrived from far away lands and left their marks which can be seen and felt even today. When it came under the Buddhists influence that lasted for many centuries it achieved high point in learning both in arts and sciences. During this period Gandhara seems to be unique among the contemporary civilisations to independently develop its own medicine and more importantly practice of surgery based on rational principles. It is a fact of history and archaeological reality that the Buddhist Gandhara was the only place in the World outside the Roman Empire where high surgical skills were acquired and put into practice. The history of art, literature and various sciences taught in the universities of Gandhara has been well documented. However the historiographers have not fully examined or talked about the available evidence that support the advancement which was achieved in medicine particularly, the corroborated evidence regarding surgery despite unequivocal archaeological verification. In this study an attempt is made to investigate the archaeological and historical evidences and evaluate how the surgery and medicine developed, progressed and then declined in Gandhara. It is important tc keep in mind that the history of medicine of any civilisation cannot be studied in isolation, since it is directly influenced by the on going social changes, cultural conflicts and upheavals and most importantly by the technological progress that the society can manage. Here we must also look at the technological progression of the people of Gandhara that enabled them to attain the advance in rational medicine and surgery during the Buddhist domination. In the chronology of events inclusion of the relevant social wax and wane and their consequences are not only inevitable but an overriding factor for better orientation the course of history. Moreover for the sake of continuity a look into the past as far back as possible is also of paramount importance.

When we look at the evolution of the health care in general terms, we notice that the human skills were evolved in a step by step manner over a long period during the evolution of human race. We are told that the major changes which took place in the development of brain size and intelligence coincided with the ability of human beings to live together in social groups.[1] Glancing through the evolution of medicine we are further informed by the medical anthropologists that the newly socialised human beings as a matter of necessity started practicing some rudimentary form of medicine and even surgery at quite early stage. The medicine man seems to be present among the earliest settlements. The anthropologists have also made a case for caring among early societies from the discovery

[1] Mithen S. *The prehistory of the mind,* London: Thames and Hudson Ltd., 1996.

and study of toothless jaw bones belonging to individuals who were incapable of biting or chewing and must have been provided suitably prepared food by others within the community. Such communal responsibilities and interdependence within the family unit offered the opportunities to man to learn how to protect the frail or weaker family members from many of the hazards faced by the primitive tribal communities. In the hostile surroundings senior and wiser clan members assumed the guardianship of the needy by protecting and looking after the very young, very old and very weak, nursing and feeding the injured and those who were ill. According to Sir William Osler (1849-1919), 'medicine arose out of the primal sympathy of man with man, out of desire to help those in sorrow, need and sicknesses'. In due course from the experience gained as a result of primordial desire of caring emerged early practice of medicine and surgery.

A study of cave paintings where several human figures seem to interact with each other have been interpreted that few individuals are helping a fellow kinsman who is in some kind of distress due to illness or injury.[2] Today huge amount of information is available in respect of paleopathology that makes it convincingly obvious that man's suffering due to injuries and infection particularly affecting the bones resulting through the struggles of surviving often required some kind of surgical intervention. The scars of the oozing sinuses due to bony infections, broken bones and many other agonising afflictions may be witnessed in human bones preserved in the museums of paleopathology. Perhaps the thinking animal early on learnt to use simple methods like rubbing, massaging and application of warmth or leaves etc. or even immobilisation simply because such a course of action offered some relief from pain. This also led to the use of primitive tools like stone knives and then surgical

---

[2] Lewis-Williams JD. *Believing and seeing: Symbolic meanings in Southern San rock paintings,* London: Academic Press, 1981, pp. 77-101.

implements made of other materials such as animal bones or suitably crafted tools from wood or other organic products.[3] During the early Iron Age metal implements were available not only as tools for day to day use in the trade and crafts but the same or similar implements must have been used for surgical purposes as well whenever such a need arose. A pair of forceps is among the earliest metal instruments ever excavated; one was discovered from Ur and considered to belong to 3200-2500 BCE.[4] It might have been part of a cosmetic box for plucking eye brows of a fashionable lady who used it as tweezers but can equally be used picking thorn or foreign bodies from the flesh as a surgical forceps. The archaeological evidence of surgery in the form of trepanation in antediluvian skulls older than 15 thousand years may be witnessed in many museums of anthropology. The argument that the holes were made in the living is no more controversial because they show growth or deposition of new bone, bearing sufficient evidence that in some cases the individuals survived long after the brutal surgery was carried out.[5] On the other hand unlike the operated skulls which have survived, the perishable soft parts of human body that might have borne the marks of operation have not survived as witness. But it is plausible that from animal husbandry people must have experienced and learnt to pluck out the unborn in the event of the death of a mother who was full term at the time of sudden accidental death. After all a caesarean section where the mother survived was only performed on a kitchen table as recently as 1793.[6] According to the Old Testament the covenant of

---

[3] Kirkup J. *The evolution of surgical instruments: An illustrated history from ancient times to the twentieth century,* Novato, California: Norman, 2005.

[4] Müller-Christensen W. *The history of the forceps,* Copenhagen and London: Humphrey Milford, Oxford University Press, 1938, p. 6.

[5] Parry TW 'Trephination of the living human skull in prehistoric times', *BMJ* 1923, vol. I, pp. 457-60.

[6] Naqvi NH. 'James Barlow (1767-1839) Operator of the first successful' caesarean section in England, *British J Obst and Gyn,* 1985; 92: 468-72.

circumcision was obediently carried out by the wife of Prophet Abraham on her own eight day old son using a flint knife. Since then this ritualistic surgery has been practiced and survived till this day as a matter of religious obligation. How the same ritual was also adopted by many tribal societies living in diverse geographic areas of the globe and never heard of Abraham or Moses, is a question the anthropologists have not yet answered satisfactorily. The operation of circumcision is also the only surgical procedure that has been discovered depicted in a frieze belonging to the Egyptian civilisation of about 5000 years.[7]

It is evident that surgery of some kind was practiced through out the known past with primitive instruments like stone knives, implements of wood, bone, and horn; without anaesthesia and with little knowledge of human body systems.[8] Hitherto surgical anaesthesia was first used only in 1845 half a century after the first maternal survival following a caesarean section. The surgical achievement of today is a great human triumph but the evolutionary process it has gone through is a story of untold pain and immeasurable human sufferings.

Medical care also seems to have evolved independently although not evenly among various civilisations. Its knowledge and its expertise have also travelled from one part of the World or from one civilisation to another even before the advent of writing. The diversity in medical care is perceptible in the development of number of medical systems over a long period of time in different parts of the World. These diverse systems also show many similarities that may be observed in the modalities of treatments practiced by the ancient medical practitioners across the globe. The early

---

[7] Nunn JF. *Ancient Egyptian Medicine,* London: British Museum Press, 1996, pp. 169-71.

[8] Neuburger M, *History of medicine,* Playfair E., tr. vol. I, London: Oxford University Press, 1910, pp. 9-10.

medical therapies were largely derived from herbal products; some of these happen to be common not only in Greek, Chinese and Ayurvedic Medicine which had historic contacts but also amongby isolated tribal societies who apparently had no contacts with each other isolated. We may assume that the observation prone mind must have independently discovered various natural therapies. Later, of course the trade among the ancients did play crucial role in the dissemination of such useful information with regard to therapies and treatments. Still later when writing became common the medical books were probably the first to travel long distances to reach the eager practitioners of far away places. The Buddhists travellers who helped to spread Buddhism to China and beyond are known to take with them medical documents along with the sacred manuscripts that were written on birch bark in the monasteries of Gandhara. The Buddhist monks who travelled from China to India have left records detailing their observations about medical and surgical knowledge, consequently transferring it between Buddhist Monasteries in Gandhara and other remote places like China. Similar exchanges were also carried out in later times by the European missionaries from China to the West. For example the French missionaries who were the first to gain access into China brought back and introduced the Chinese medicine to their Western colleagues who were particularly fascinated by the Chinese diagnostic skills by palpation. One of the earliest translations of the Chinese medical textbook was carried out by a French missionary, Father Michael Boym (1612-1659 CE) who was known to have translated one of the Chinese texts on the examination of the pulse called *Maijing* in to Latin in 1852 and the same was translated into French in 1671. In 1682 Boym's work was translated into other languages thus introducing the Chinese method of examination of the pulse to other parts of Europe. It was Sir John Floyer, who in 1707 introduced the first watch with a hand that can run for one minute during which the pulse may be counted accurately during a unit time. Introduction of such a watch ensured counting the pulse rate per minute as the universal clinical examination and the watch a symbol for the physicians. It is known that Sir John Floyer possessed an English translation of *Maijing.*[9]

In view of the remoteness of the period and dearth of documented data with regard to medicine and surgery practiced by Buddhists of Gandhara, the emphasis would be to bring into discussion as many available historiographical sources as possible. This is necessary in order to collate and analyse many accessible accounts however limited information they might contain. There is no doubt that a broader discussion is essential because as pointed out above the subject has hardly been examined before and not many pertinent references can be put together to make a pivotal points from where any logical dialogue may set in motion. The greater emphasis is on the archaeological artefacts that are now established to be the surgical instruments discovered in Taxila and other places that were part of old Gandhara. Their discovery is highly significant because Taxila remained the capital of Gandhara through out the ancient times and social historians unanimously agree that it was known as an important centre for education in art and all sciences. Its reputation during the antiquity as a centre of excellence for medical teaching was known in far off places.[10] Royalties, rich people and poor all liked to send their sons to be taught by the renowned teachers who dwelled in Taxila. Among these teachers were physicians and surgeons. Being a large city that was religious and political capital for centuries Taxila must have all kind of medical and surgical services for its population.

---

[9] Floyer J. *The physician's pulse watch: or, an essay to explain the old art of feeling the pulse, and to improve it by the help. Of pulse watch...to which is added an extract out of Andrew Cleyer, concerning the Chinese art of feeling the pulse,* London: S. Smith and B. Walford, J. Nicholson, 1707-10.

[10] Mookerji RK. *Ancient Indian education,* London: Macmillan and Co. Limited, 1947, p. 470.

There are few imperative factors listed below that guide us towards the conclusion that discovery of surgical instruments from Taxila and few other sites in Gandhara was not in any way a surprise find.

The inhabitants of Gandhara were skilful in metallurgy, a fact comes home so obviously from the multitudes of fine metal objects excavated related to arts, domestic use and for trades. The quality in design and purity of metals these are made is remarkable for the period. Also the same supposition can be confirmed from the continuously improved quality of coinage as with other metal objects. The evidence of metallurgical skills of the ancients is apparent from the quality of the inscribed iron pillars still standing from the time of Ashoka. Similarly the weight of the silver coin from the Mauryan period was same as the smallest standardised unit of weight from the Indus Valley Civilisation and was still in use during modern times.

The tradition of medical education during ancient times in Taxila is well proven on sound historical grounds. It was natural that progress in surgery and instrumentation would also take place in a centre that was famous for medical teaching.

There is evidence that a rational and compassionate form of Buddhism was evolved in Gandhara which influenced the monasteries to become centre of medical service for the people. Some of these monasteries also provided surgical treatment whenever required thus offering a free comprehensive caring medical service.

The history of Gandhara as summarised below shows that for centuries it was a melting pot of civilisations offering opportunities for the evolution of ideas. It was the first land which the Aryans populated during their migration, bringing their own social, cultural and liturgical traditions. Long after Aryans, a prevailing wave of Persian was followed by Greeks and many more came and went or choose to settle in

Gandhara. All contributed in its communal matrix, the Buddhists probably gave more in terms of art, religious and social life. The evidence of their medical and surgical contributions no doubt is most visible and subject of analysis in the forthcoming pages.

The compelling religious symbols still seen in numerous monasteries, stone images or rock carvings in most remote mountain passes, all tell stories about the human struggle not just against the elements but also against natural disasters and diseases. Among these icons we must add the surgical instruments and many other medical objects with which they tried to fight the illness.

There is also great deal of evidence about the part people of Gandhara played in the progress of Ayurvedic system of medicine. In fact it might be true that Gandhara was the birth place of Ayurvedic system and the word Ayurveda was first used in *Caraka Samhita,* which is universally accepted to be written in Gandhara.

A number of important rulers such as Kanishka, whose reign lasted for a long time and his royal patronage to the art and science, are well documented further adding to the fact that whenever right environment prevailed in Gandhara it brought progress and prosperity.

Apart from the surgical instruments the discovery of well preserved apparatus like condensers and a scientific system of weights and measurements also gives convincing evidence for the growth of rational thinking.

Since Gandhara was the first station which attracted the migrating Aryans, where they had their very first settlements and the new comers also compiled their first writings after settling in this area. They were followed over the centuries by others. Similarly it is also highly plausible from the chronology that the medical texts along with other pedagogic writings were first originated in the region of Gandhara and from here the medical knowledge contained in them and taught in the schools of Gandhara was transmitted to other places.

The cultivation of medicinal plants and importing those not found in the region is well documented on some of the stone edicts from the time of Ashoka. Taxila was his favourite place where Ashoka was governor during the reign of his father. There are various historical indications that all kinds of herbs were found in the surrounding hills around Taxila. Many of the archaeological objects discovered in Taxila may indicate that it also developed into a centre for the cultivation of medicinal plants and producing medicines from herbal and non herbal sources.

1.
A brief history of Gandhara

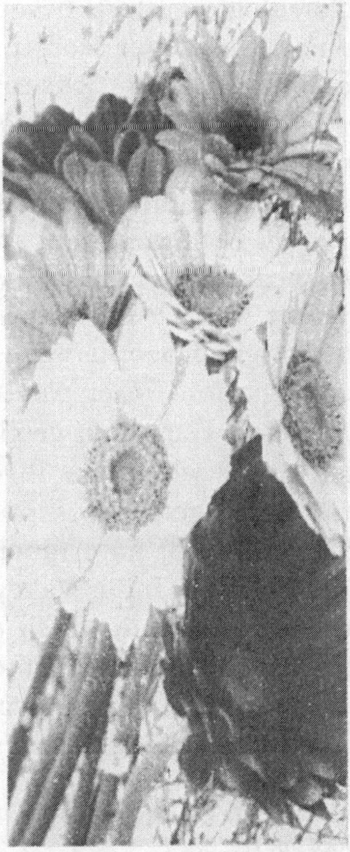

The history of Gandhara can be traced from the Neolithic period, even though the excavations that have revealed material from the Stone Age have been carried out only in a limited area. But few objects that have been discovered offer enough evidence of the settlements going back to Stone Age. Although at currently there is reduced archaeological and enough archaeological efforts have yet not been made. But there is sufficient evidence from previous excavations that shows earliest human presence in Gandhara. Nonetheless even the limited archaeological discoveries of recent period have exposed at least two major sites where Stone Age tools, bones of hunted animals and other objects have been discovered. Both these sites are in Gandhara, one is the set of caves near city of Mardan while the other is in the hills surrounding Taxila.[11] But very little is known about Gandhara and its original people who inhabited this area before the Aryan migration. When we look for the contacts between Gandhara and Harappan civilisation; we discover that the archaeologists who were involved in the early excavations in Gandhara generally supported the view that pre-Vedic Gandhara did not have much contacts with the Harappan civilisation of the Indus Valley. However recently a diverse opinion has emerged, which argues in favour of decipherable contacts indicating some influence of the Harappan civilisation over Gandhara.[12] May be future excavations might tell us more about the people of pre-

[11] Dani AH. *The historic city of Taxila,* Tokyo: The Centre for East Asian Cultural Studies, 1986, pp. 18-28.

[12] Agrawal A, ed., *In search of Vedic-Harappan relationship,* New Delhi: Aryan Books International, 2005.

history who inhabited this region and how their contacts developed with neighbouring civilisations in the North and South.

From the study based on the objects and other implements that have been excavated at a number of sites belonging to the Neolithic period, there is plentiful substantiation that Gandhara was an agricultural based society.

Some times after second half of second millennium BCE this land was flooded by the greatest migration of people this World has ever seen, it was the Indo-European people who started their movement into South Asia, historians have given them the name of Aryans. The Aryans from the North migrated in huge numbers crossing the rivers and mountainous passes and made their first permanent settlements in this land that in their writings was first described as Gandhara. Once they settled down in the land of their choice tthey started to evolve their own traditions, social customs and liturgy. One custom they brought with them or adopted during the migration was sacrifice of animals which, lasted in their society for a long time. The overwhelming numbers and their well organised community setup simply inundated the indigenous population the fate of which remains unknown. They might have assimilated or perished or dispersed into oblivion. Once the generations of newcomers settled they gradually established a code of conduct for their society. The priests created and memorised the literature that is now known as *Vedas* meaning knowledge. The earliest known to us and even available today is called *Rig-Veda.* It is difficult to date its origins, however it must be accumulated over a long period of time that might be earlier or around 1000 BCE. For centuries it passed in the form of oral traditions from one priest to another or father to son and at an unknown date it was ultimately compiled in written form. So what we have today might be unrecognisable to those who used to memorise it in earlier times. The huge tom comprising of 1028 hymns does not tell any stories of human triumph or narrates any form of chronology or even primarily lays down laws but is dedicated to eulogize superlatively hymns in praise of gods. Among these gods Agni is one of the greatest, who perhaps has more hymns dedicated than any other god mentioned in *Rig-Veda.* This also furnishes some hint that conceivably both Zoroastrian and Vedics religions might have branched off from single parent religion prior to the migration of both into their respective new lands of Persia and Gandhara. In *Rig-Veda* the earliest eight settlements of Vedic period are mentioned and Gandhara is the very first on the list. The commentators have interpreted the geographical position of Vedic Gandhara in relation to the river Kabul (*Kubha* in Sanskrit) and the river Indus. This relationship fairly accurately puts the region of Gandhara in the position where it existed in real during its later geographical location. Apart from a settlement with the name of Gandhara there is also mention of a tribe with the name of Gandhari. Yet one more entity derived from Gandhara that has been mentioned many times in the *Rig-Veda* is Gandharva. In a number of hymns, an example is quoted below Gandharva is alluded to in a spiritual or celestial context.[13]

> This steed which Yama gave hath Trita harnessed, and him the first of all, hath Indra mounted. His bridle the Gandharva grasped.
>
> Book I. Hymn CLXIII, 2. The Horse.

The expert of Sanskrit language may argue the fine differences between Gandharva mentioned in the above verse and Gandhari depicted in other verses of *Rig-Veda,* but the word Gandharva has been interpreted in the notes of the translator as 'heavenly beings that dwell in the region of air and guard the sacred soma'. Gandharvas were also

---

[13] Griffith RTH. tr., *The hymns of the Rigveda,* Benares: E J Lazarus and Co., 1920.

divine singers of hymns. While according to a post Vedic text known as *Gandharva Samhita* dealing with music, the third note of the Indian music scale '*ga*' is a shortened version of Gandharva. There is also some evidence that physicians were also called Gandharvas and after about 13th century CE when the pulse examination was established in Ayurvedic Medicine, a pulse was named Gandharvi.[14] Further still others have inferred that Gandharvas are simply those who were the inhabitants of Gandhara.

However it is not possible to place Gandhara on a definite time line owing to many historical incongruities in Indian history. In this respect we are not able to reach any final satisfactory conclusion because the ancient Indians though had contributed to all forms of literature narrating of history was undoubtedly singularly absent from their writings and they have left no accounts of historiography at all.[15] The veracity of poverty in recording the chronology is well recognized and accepted by all renowned historians of modern times.[16] As an example there is no mention of Alexander's invasion in any Indian writing is sufficient evidence to this well acknowledged viewpoint. The first person to write Indian history after living in India for many years was Abu Rihan Alberuni (973-1048 CE) who had complete understanding of Sanskrit and also had access to many Sanskrit texts that have not survived today. Alberuni has mentioned Gandhara (Alqandhar in Arabic) and during his time its capital was Vaihand or Ohind, which still exists on the right bank of the river Indus with slight variation of its name. He also confirms by referring the school of *Samkhya* philosophy that Gandharvas belonged to the spiritual beings,

---

[14] Meulenbeld GJ. *A history of Indian medical literature*, vol. II A, Groningen: Egbert Forsten, 2000, pp. 427-28.

[15] Sastri G. *A concise history of classical Sanskrit literature*, London: Oxford University Press, 1960, pp. 126-29.

[16] Thapar R. *Ancient Indian social history: some interpretations*, Delhi: Sangam Books, 1996, p. 237.

while in another place Alberuni reflecting on to the *Rig-Veda* tells us that Gandharvas were musicians and singers to the Devas or gods.[17]

It may be that during early Vedic period Gandhara was a divinely blissful mythical place, with time became a reality on the earth due to the environmental attractiveness of the region. Considering the abundance of natural resources, high mountains, streams flowing with sweet water and the great rivers; the region was able to sustain a bewildering variety of animal and plant life, no wonder the Aryan settlers considered it a heaven. As the fate has it in reality this heaven on earth is also sitting on the most unstable and greatest fault line on the earth. This irony made the idyllic heaven also the most dangerous place to live which has suffered frequent devastating earthquakes that have been a consistent feature throughout the history. The archaeologists have discovered widespread damage caused by earthquakes to many of the ancient buildings after these structures were unearthed. A recent earthquake on October 8, 2005 killed nearly hundred thousands people, and demolished virtually every building with in a vast area, leaving many millions without shelter. Such disasters have happened regularly both in the recent past and in remote past leaving their scars that may be witnessed even today.

Reverting back to our topic it is important to look critically as regard to the concepts of surgery in *Rig-Veda,* a subject of immense din and claims recorded in numerous publications. Some of the hymns in *Rig-Veda* allude to amputation of legs and new limbs have been surgically grafted, eyes enucleated and replaced and also grafting the animal heads on to the trunks of humans. All such feats are confined to the realm of mysticism or miracles performed by gods for other gods. In the narratives these procedures

[17] Alberuni. *Alberuni's India,* Sachau EC, ed. and tr., New Delhi: Atlantic Publishers and Distributors, 1989, pp. 89, 259.

were not carried out on the earth for earthly beings. The hymns of *Rig-Veda* also mentions mythical treatments and hymns are recited in honour of gods who performed them. As examples the twin brother gods known as Asvins in *Rig-Veda* are admired as *Bhaishaja* or physicians to the other gods. Their admiration for performing miraculous medical and surgical feats is restricted exclusively in the realm of supernatural. On the other hand the same Asvins are also despised in hymns by some gods for their involvement in such acts.

The post-Vedic literature generally referred as *Dharma* literature has also loathed physicians as low creatures and categorized them as unclean. In ancient Indian literature this love hate relationship with the practitioners of medicine and surgery is utterly perplexing for those happen to study the history of medicine during remote antiquity.

With regard to Gandhara no controversy is present in the sacred books belonging to later period such as *Ramayana* (500 BCE to 100 BCE) and *Mahabharata* (400 BCE to 400 CE), both these epics unambiguously recognise Gandhara a country and mention Takshashila or Taxila as the capital of Gandhara. In *Mahabharata* Gandhari was the princess from Gandhara who was married to the blind king of the Kurus. In current local language Gandhari is also a garment made from the wool of the sheep found in the mountains of the region. The name of south eastern province in Afghanistan and its capital Kandahar or Qandahar is what remains today as a relic from the past. Still the borders of Gandhara were never defined and always remained fluid. Whenever a strong and powerful monarch ruled the borders were extended but reduced when centre became weak and feeble.

More recently scholars working on some of the newly acquired Birch Bark scrolls have named the language Gandhari, a new name of the old language that previous historians had recorded as Prakrit written in Kharoshthi script that was adapted from Aramaic. It was the day to day language based on Sanskrit but spoken and used for the written literature in Gandhara.

Leaving aside the mythology and legends the history has recorded that Cyrus (590-529 BCE) conquered Gandhara in about 530 BCE. On an inscription at the tomb of Darius (550-486 BCE) the name Gandhara appears as Gadara. In the ruins of Persepolis in Iran the great marble stair case leading to the palace is decorated with figures of the people from all corners of the empire bringing their gifts to the king of kings, where presence of a Gandharian is noticeable.[18] In *The Histories,* Herodotus (490 BCE) has referred the area surrounding the present day Peshawar as Paktuike. The name referred by Herodotus is intriguing because it resonates even to this day; a large part of today's Gandhara is inhabited by Pakhtun speaking people in area that includes present day Paktiya in Afghanistan and along the Pakistan-Afghanistan border in Pakistan. Herodotus further informs us that Gandhara was the 20th richest province in the Achaemenian Empire during the reign of Darius and also provided a contingent to fight along with his army against the Greeks.[19] The area has been the arena where great political games have been played for centuries. what Rudyard Kipling has written with the relish and delight of a true imperialist in his famous story of *Kim* about the race for dominance of this land among the competing colonial powers of Russia and Britain. Even though the people of this land are among the poorest and the rugged mountains lack any wealth such as oil, still even in modern times the British, Russians and now the neo-colonist US all have sent their armies into this region only to leave after

---

[18] Ghani F. *Archaeological site in Faras (Perspolis),* Tehran: Yassavoli Publications, 1998, pp. 50-55.

[19] Herodotus. *The Histories* (Book 3), Grene D, tr., Chicago: University of Chicago Press, 1987, p. 94.

futile slaughter and destruction. It is obvious that history is a very poor teacher.

The Achaemenian conquest brought revolutionary transformations affecting the inhabitants throughout the vast region of Gandhara. The most important impact was due to the migration of diverse people from Persia, Greece and even China. Before the conquest Darius had assigned his Greek admiral Scylax to map out a water route along the river Indus that opened another door for strange looking outsiders reaching Gandhara from far away places.[20] The trade with Rome prospered and more dry trade routes which afterwards were famously known as Silk Road were established. The Gandhara art and literature was heavily influenced and Taxila emerged as the centre of learning of all sciences. On the other hand the cast system which by now was deeply rooted among the descendants of Aryan migrants, resentfully detested mixing with people of different colour or creed and the presence of unclean foreigners was to them repugnant and intolerable. Many chose to move further South to live in the heaven of the pure in the cities that were emerging on the banks of sacred waters of the rivers Yamuna and Ganges to live in a social structure controlled by those of high cast. The deep rooted hatred for each other amongst the inhabitants living in the North and those living in the South was reciprocal and long lasting. The literature of the time offers glimpses where those living in the Ganges plains considered the Northern unclean so much so that even to touch them was an act of sin. In his book, *a history of India,* the author, R. Thapar portrays an interesting contrast highlighting the degree of hostility between the South and North in these words.[21]

---

[20] Dunbar G. *A history of India from the earliest times to the present day,* London: Nicholson and Watson Limited, 1943, p. 29.

[21] Thapar R. *A history of India,* vol. I, London: Penguin Books, 1966, pp. 59-60.

> The more orthodox Brahmans treated this region (Gandhara) as impure since it had come under Persian domination. It would appear that a number of non-Aryan practices were still prevalent in north-western India. Orthodox Aryanism had spread eastwards, leaving the north-west open to contend with the foreigners who were regarded as impure.

An equally converse acidic vision reciprocating opposite contempt may be observed in the texts written in the North. An example may be found in the *Caraka Samhita* itself against the people living in the South. They are belittled by derogatory names as Dravidas and Andhrakas. Such a muted projection has been alleged by a modern historian of history of Indian science Debiprasad Chattopadhyaya, was owing to the Kashmiri background of the final compiler of the *Caraka Samhita*. The degree of acrimonious resentment may be judged by the following quote of the above author from *Caraka Samhita*.[22]

> *Caraka Samhita* V.5.29: Seeing these persons in dreams is supposed to be as ominous as dreaming the dogs, demons and untouchables, etc.

At the time when Achaemenid Empire had reached its glory and had a complete control over Gandhara there were two great movements in India. It is speculated by some historians that it was a result of reaction from perpetual oppressing hold of the high cast Brahmanism over society. Jainism pioneered by Mahavira (599-527 BCE) remained limited and at the periphery of Hinduism. On the other hand the Buddhism preached by Buddha (562-480 BCE) proved more dynamic, spreading rapidly far beyond the borders of India and breaking off completely from the mother religion.[23] When it reached Gandhara it prospered and not only dominated for centuries but also spread to

---

[22] Chattopadhyaya D. *Science and society in ancient India*, Calcutta: Research India Publications, 1977, p. 31.

[23] Armstrong K. *Buddha*, London: Weidenfeld and Nicholson, 2000. See

Central Asia, China, Korea, and Japan by the travellers whose enthusiasm must be greatly fired by their religious zeal making gigantic efforts to walking through the treacherous snow clad mountain passes and most hazardous deserts in order to spread Buddha's message. Many of these Buddhist missionaries travelled from Gandhara, crossing the difficult mountains, passing through the Gobi desert taking the message to the remote corners of the earth. In late 19th to early 20th century this area became centre for the race among the Western collectors of Buddhist antiquities, who have now been dubbed as foreign devils.[24] It is most unfortunate that the bulk of the hoards of antiquities they made so much effort to find are still stored in original boxes and not yet freed to researchers. Among the manuscripts they collected, few were medical texts that will be discussed later but no surgical instruments or any other medical artifacts were included among their varied finds from the deserts or the Silk Road. The neo-travellers have left their marks still visible in their writings describing the harsh experiences during their wanderings in the 'mountains of gods' and inhospitable deserts, in the foot steps of the Chinese travellers who traversed this region during the ancient times.

The whirlwind campaign of Alexander the great and his grand welcome during the short stay in Taxila in 326 BCE did no damage to Buddhism. On the other hand Alexander's quick exit helped to strengthen the ties with the Greek civilization. Even prior to Alexander there was a long history of contacts with the Greeks.[25] The post-Alexander Greek influence is the most critical and remarkable episode in the history of Gandhara. Although in one aspect it is extraordinary that the superior Greek

---

also Bechert H, ed., *The dating of the historical Buddha*, Gottingen: Vandenhoeck and Ruprecht, 1991.

[24] Hop Kirk P. *Foreign devils on the Silk Road: The search for the lost treasurers of central Asia*, Oxford: Oxford University Press, 1980.

[25] Narain AK. *The Indo-Greeks*, Oxford: The Clarendon Press, 1957.

learning was readily adopted by all those who were conquered and came into the fold or its sway, but on the other hand the conquered people were not influenced by the Greek polytheistic tendencies. It is also true that these invaders of Gandhara seem to be always eager to discard their own creed and readily convert whenever they came in contact with the strong religious force. As an example almost all new comers despite the fact they came as conquerors in Gandhara speedily adopted Buddhism becoming most ardent servants of Buddha, despite they had followed the Greek pantheon for a considerable long period. But the Greek art they bought had a strong impact on Gandhara's Buddhist art and sculpture, an important topic discussed at great lengths by many authors. A classical in depth study in this respect was carried out by the French archaeologist, illustrating the Greek influence from the Gandhara sculptures, some he himself helped to unearth at different sites.[26] The image of the head of a Gandhara sculpture in the first figure presents a typical and convincing example where Greek influence on Gandhara art is clearly noticeable (Fig.1). Similar influence may be seen in numerous other sculptures exhibited in most museums in India or Pakistan and almost all major museums in the World, where the pieces of Gandhara sculptures were transported legally or illegally after their discovery. From the time the discoveries were made till now some of the best specimens were mostly illegally removed and are in private collections in the West making valuable investment, occasionally coming into international art market. Same is applied to other articles including coins, jewellery, terracotta, and metal artefacts although no surgical instrument of Gandhara origin has ever been spotted in a market place or in private collections. Perhaps the traders in art were not interested in the less glamorous pieces of metal, which were not even recognisable or had no investment value. It may also be true that there was no big

[26] Faucher A. *L'Art Gréco-Bouddhique du Gandhâra*, Paris: Imprimerie Nationale, 1905.

demand for such items in the international market and these low-key antiquities were not sought out by many collectors.

Nonetheless some of the excavated items now confirmed as surgical instruments can only be seen in the Taxila Museum and no other museum seems to hold the surgical instruments or medically related objects that can be compared with similar objects or with the excavated surgical instruments from Greek and Roman period.

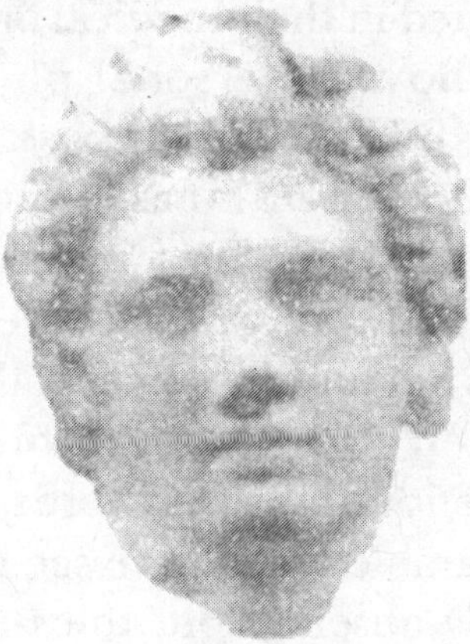

Fig. 1

Head of Gandhara sculpture presenting a fine example of Greek influence.
(Image courtesy of www.gandhara.com.au)

One perplexing feature regarding the Greek influence on Gandhara is that it is so dynamically noticeable in the art but almost non-existence on other important aspects of social life of the people as we see from the artefacts and historical texts. Whatever we know of the early social history of medicine in Gandhara the Greek empirical or experiential notions in medicine did not make any impact on the Gandhara medicine. The well established traditions of experiments in physiology or methodical study of the human anatomy through dissection was well established in Greek traditions, but these were not exported in the same way as we see its influence on the sculpture and art. We notice a strange anomaly regarding a robust Greek influence on the art of

Gandhara but no impact at all on other social aspects such as medicine. The medicine in Gandhara, where contacts with Greek civilizations were so close and prolonged remained free from such influences. For example medical men in Gandhara never discovered Hippocrates, Herophilus or even the Roman surgeon Celsus or Galen who were in reality their contemporary. The diagnostics of Greek medicine was based on elaborate pulse lore, which was known to be taught from the time of Praxagoras (4th century BCE) and was strongly rooted in their medical practice by physician like Erasistratus, who was personal physician to Selucus Nicator I (358-281 BCE). The ambassador of Nicator I, Megasthenes (350-250 BCE) himself had great interest in medicine and stayed in India for a long time, also wrote the first history of India known as *Indica.* Despite these strong and positive contacts no Buddhist or any other Indian medical text ever mentioned the examination of the pulse or physiology of circulation. In other words clinical diagnostic methodology comparable to what we see in Greek medicine is seemingly entirely absent from the Indian medicine of the contemporary period. Such an analysis is further reinforced and underpinned by the following quote from Kutambiah.[27]

> Caraka belongs to the second century AD and if he had borrowed anything from the medicine of the Greeks of his time, certainly one would think that the pulse lore would have been the first. As matter of fact, pulse lore is not mentioned in the ancient medical classics of Caraka and Susruta. It finds it way into Indian medicine (only) in the 13th century AD.

When we look at the design of surgical instruments and other associated artefacts we find that it also remained strictly local without any influence from the Greek conquerors. Although many of these objects were excavated from a city planned by the Greek town planners built on grid pattern.

[27] Kutambiah P. *Ancient Indian medicine,* Bombay: Orient Longman, 1962, p. xlii.

It is also extraordinary that Gandhara has not yielded any Greek or Roman style instruments but only locally crafted typical Buddhist instruments have been discovered. A selective and discerning impact that is notably seen in the sculptures, coins and few other areas of art is totally absent in medical artefacts. This interesting realism deserved to be analysed fully. The presence of Greek artisans in Gandhara is as visible as the absence of Greek physicians.

The first golden age in the history of Gandhara started soon after Alexander died and Gandhara finally came in to Mauryan control in about 305 BCE. After Ashoka succeeded to Mauryan throne and also converted to Buddhism he made Taxila capital of Gandhara and the centre of Buddhism. It is understandable why Ashoka had special fondness for Gandhara and its capital. He had made it a seat of scholars when he served as the governor of Gandhara during the reign of his father Bindusara or probably his grandfather Chandragupta. The largest Stupa in Taxila called Dharmarajika Stupa was originally built by Ashoka after he ascended to the throne. In this Stupa he had also installed the sacred relics of Buddha's bones. The Stupa was probably extended or rebuilt during the reign of Kanishka who was equally enthusiastic follower of Buddhism. There is another famous Stupa in Taxila known as Kunala Stupa which is associated with the legend related to the son of Ashoka whose name was Kunala and also served as governor of Gandhara under his father. Ashoka has left potent symbols of his compassionate long rule in the form of inscriptions or edicts written in Greek, Pali, Kharoshthi and other languages in all corners of his vast kingdom. In all 33 edicts written on stone or iron pillars have been discovered, some of these were also erected in Gandhara and present to this day. All these edicts were erected after Ashoka gave up the life of conquests and blood shedding and had adopted Buddhism. After this transformation he embarked on many projects of charities and considered the people his children. The theme etched on the edicts was chiefly influenced from his religious zeal to emulate the teachings of Buddha. Most of the edicts were not for the glorification or his personal gratification or even strictly religious propaganda of Buddhism but most of the edicts inform the public about the social welfare works in his kingdoms. The inscription quoted below is a good example of his compassion and genuine intension to do good for the poor. The inscription informs the people about establishing a kind of a free health service in his empire not only for humans but for animals as well; this must be the unique first recorded example in the history of humanity.[28]

> Everywhere within, Beloved-of-the-Gods, King Piyadasi's domain, and among the people beyond the borders, the Cholas, the Pandyas, the Satiyaputras, the Keralaputras, as far as Tamraparni and where the Greek king Antiochos rules, and among the kings who are eighbours of Antiochos, everywhere has Beloved-of-the-Gods, King Piyadasi, made provision for two types of medical treatment: medical treatment for humans and medical treatment for animals. Wherever medical herbs suitable for humans or animals are not available, I have had them imported and grown. Wherever medical roots or fruits are not available I have had them imported and grown. Along roads I have had wells dug and trees planted for the benefit of humans and animals

Asoka's other great contribution for the cause of Buddhism was calling the third Buddhist Council in 250 BCE to iron out some differences that had crept into the faith and thus strengthened the faith he was so passionate about. On political front too Ashoka made the empire strong during his life time and most importantly acquired genuine popularity and true love of his people, particularly the people of Gandhara. Ashoka who ruled from 273 to 232 BCE in his own persona evidently symbolized strong influence of Greek culture. According to some historians his mother was daughter or niece of Selucus Nicator I, given

[28] Sircar DC. *Inscriptions of Ashoka*, Delhi: South Asia Books, Second edition, 1998.

in marriage to conclude the peace treaty. In return Selucus Nicator received 500 elephants which he desperately needed to strengthen his army to keep control of Asia Minor.

Strangely enough after Ashoka's death the Mauryan Empire quickly disintegrated and Gandhara came in to the control of new bread generally known as Indo-Greeks who had gained the control in Asia Minor after freeing themselves from the yolk of Seleucids and entered Gandhara for which they always had a longing to regain control. Menander a soldier scholar most probably ruled between 180-160 BCE becoming a powerful force and also adopted Buddhism. He controlled not just Gandhara but whole of Punjab and made incursions further into the Ganges plains. The strength and sway during his time in Gandhara may be judged from the Greek new city in Taxila which Menander founded and called it Sirkap. As mentioned above it was laid on a plan of a typical Greek metropolis built on grid pattern and has been completely excavated; a number of surgical instruments that are to be discussed later were discovered from this site.

The chronology of Gandhara between 200 BCE to the invasion of white Huns in fifth century CE had posed many difficulties to the historians due to numerous missing links because a number of dynasties came and went after only very short rules. But most of the confusion has been more or less resolved from the dates inscribed on the coins, which have been discovered as a result of recent excavations, these coins have helped a great deal in filling the gaps. This confusion can be noticed if one is reading a historical account written before the first half of twentieth century and those written after the new discoveries that have thrown fresh light on the past events. The coins also clarified the identities of various invaders, from Central Asia who defeated the Greeks in Bactria and gradually advanced to occupy Gandhara. The first wave is known as Sakas and Scythians who to start with were all nomadic people but were civilized by Greek influence and culture, when they came in contact with

Buddhism in Gandhara they were converted to Buddhism serving it obsessively. During middle of first century CE yet another invasion by Kushans who had their origin from further North in Central Asia and had controlled Bactria and Persia for long time eventually dislodged all others from Gandhara and occupied it.

The third king in the dynasty of Kushans was Kanishka, his reign marks the most important period in the history of Buddhism and the events that occurred not only in Gandhara but far beyond as well. The date of Kanishka has been the most controversial and hotly discussed topic among the historians in recent times. John Marshall (1876-1958 and later Sir John Marshall) in an early paper based on the study of coins set the date of Kanishka's accession 'close of the first century AD or later'.[29] Then in 1965 there was a debate to reach a consensus among the historians.[30] It is now agreed that Kanishka ascended to throne in about 100 CE and ruled till about 128 CE. After Ashoka his reign brought about the second golden age in the valleys and mountains of Gandhara. He made present Peshawar his capital and extended his control not just in India as far as Bengal in east and the Southern most corners to present Sri Lanka but well into Eastern China and all of Bactria. In this sense his empire was greater than even Ashoka's. The prosperity during his reign can be judged fromby the heavy and high quality gold coins issued from his mints and are displayed in the British Museum. After his conversion to Buddhism Kanishka turned out to be the most devoted Buddhist emperor after Ashoka and served the faith with sincere and competent dedication. Following in the foot steps of Ashoka he ordered the 4th Buddhist Council to be held in Kashmir which although

---

[29] Marshall JH. 'The date of Kanishka', *Journal of the Royal Asiatic Society of Great Britain and Ireland,* 1914, pp. 973-86.

[30] Ray P, Gupta HN. 'The chronology committee of the National Institute of sciences of India', *Proceedings of the chronology committee of the National Institute of sciences of India,* CHSI, 1965; 3 : pp. 223-24.

became highly controversial so much so that it was never recognized by some of the Southern Buddhist scholars. Despite the opposition Kanishka using his enormous clout strengthened the Buddhism which then spread from Gandhara to China, Korea and reached to Japan. He encouraged scholarship and dialogue among the scholars who had flocked in his court from far and wide. As a result the Buddhism that was fostered in Gandhara and had absorbed new ideas from Greek and Persian culture started to spread from Gandhara to far away places. Consequently it also emerged more rational more tolerant more compassionate and sponsor of both religious and secular learning. We may also say that the 4th Buddhist Council initiated the ethical approach that in due course had strong influence and emerged as Mahayana (Greater Vehicle) form of Buddhism. It was the result of teachings of some of the greatest philosophers of the time in the court of King Kanishka, one of them was known as Nagarjuna.[31] As a consequence a new wisdom was established and pressed forward a perception that by living with and serving the people was far better way to achieve enlightenment than austere living in isolation and inflicting self punishment in seclusion away from the people. The notion cannot be better elucidated by the story of Buddha himself, when after crossing the river by boat he met a smug ascetic who boasted that after meditating by standing in the river for fourteen years he is able to cross the river by walking on the water. Buddha responded that he did not have fourteen years to spare so he paid the boatman, who helped him cross the river and earned living for his family.

The Gandhara sculptures are known for their serene appearance and highly natural composition; they have well proportioned body and radiating face, this excellence of Gandhara sculptures was obviously due to the Greek

---

[31] Basham AL. *The wonder that was India,* London: Sidgwick and Jackson, 1967, p. 264.

influence. It was Mahayana Buddhism that patronised such an art form and placed it virtually in every nook and corner of Gandhara. In contrast as an example the Buddhist sculpture created in Tibet with grotesque shapes and contorted features were influenced by the pre-Buddhist shamanistic culture. The impact of this culture may also be seen and strongly reflected on the Tibetan medicine as well, it remains so till this date.

Although Kanishka made his administrative capital at Peshawar his spiritual attachment with Taxila was very strong where he also laid down a new city only a short distance from the old Greco-Bactrian city of Sirkap and called it Sirsukh. Long before Kanishka, Taxila had for centuries enjoyed a reputation comparable to a present day famous university town. The sponsorship and patronisation of Kanishka enhanced this image bringing not only many learned religious personalities but many teachers of secular sciences as well. Among them was Caraka who was the royal physician and also compiled *Caraka Samhita* in Taxila. The other noteworthy name already came across above was Nagarjuna who was the redactor of *Susruta Samhita.*

During the early excavations in Gandhara a historically important and most sacred relic known as Kanishka's Casket was discovered from the relic temple (*Vihara*) that was erected by Kanishka and was unearthed near Peshawar in 1909. Inside this casket was a crystal reliquary containing three small pieces of Buddha's bones. In 1910 the bones were gifted to the Buddhists of Burma by the then British colonial government.[32] Today this sacred relic attracts huge numbers of pilgrims and tourists to the temple in Mandalay. The original casket which contained this historical and sacred relic was photographed by the author during the visit at

---

[32] Cumming J Sir. *Revealing India's past, a co-operative record of archaeological conservation and exploration in India and beyond,* London: The India Society, 1939, p, 141.

Peshawar museum (Fig.2), where it is exhibited inconspicuously on the lowest shelf inside a wall cabinet without any label. Its replica can also be seen in British Museum. The circular casket is made of gilt bronze and approximately measures 20 inches in height. It is in two parts, the round lid that can be separated is decorated with carvings of lotus flower with ten petals spread out on its top. In the centre of the lid is the figure of seated Buddha with a large halo and each side are two standing figures with smaller halo, these have been described by some as Indra and Brahma. The lip of the lid that fits over to the main receptacle is more than two inches wide and decorated with swans with spread out wings, these swans are carrying a garland in their beaks. The body of the casket through out its circumference is decorated with a large drape of flowers or wreath carried by a number of figures. The central or prominent among these figures can undoubtedly be recognised as King Kanishka in his familiar dress as seen on the coins of his era and the sculptures. In side the casket a Kharoshthi inscription confirms the fact that relic was placed and dedicated by Kanishka himself. The end of the inscription bears the signature of its creator that reads, *'Servant, Agesilas, overseer of the Vihara of Kanishka'*. This undoubtedly makes it an Indo-Greek workmanship offering evidence of the Greek influence in projects relating to major works of art and architecture in Gandhara even up to the first century CE.

The era of Kanishka and his immediate successors is of greater relevance to the discussion, especially as regard the social and cultural developments throughout the Gandhara society and its prolonged impact. The benevolent regime also brought up many social changes or benefits for people such as improvements in medical care. The surgical instruments that have been discovered and were used by the Buddhist surgeons of this period offer substantial evidence of the progress not only in religious aspects but in social matters as well. In other words these implements offer forceful evidence of some kind of health care available to the people in Gandhara. The improved surgical instrumentation is also a sure indication that the users of these instruments were rational, progressive, compassionate working in a stable society.

The decline of Kushans started after about two centuries of Kushan rule, first they were ousted from the Bactria by the rising power of Sassanid dynasty of Persia in about 240 CE and over a short period they also lost their seat at Gandhara. However the remnant of Kushans survived in the form of smaller city states in some areas where they found opportunities to subdue and keep their control. The final demise started during the middle of fifth century CE when another invasion by the most aggressive and belligerent hordes from central Asia invaded Gandhara. Their origin has been a hotly discussed subject among the historians and not yet settled to the satisfaction of all. These destroyers of Gandhara are known by different names, the Byzantine historians called them Hephthalites or Ephthalites but they are commonly named as White Huns. They have also been described descendents of Hsiung-Nu tribes from the Eastern China, though it is not a convincing presumption because those who are known to be their descendents do not carry Mongol feature. This mysterious race had first overwhelmed the central Asia and controlled much of the region known as Parthia as well the eastern Persian territories for a long period. When they were dislodged from Persia by the rising Sassanid power, they entered Gandhara. This happened about the same time as the invasion of Roman Empire by the Huns of Attila. It is agreed that both these invaders had no common roots though one thing is certain that the destruction and blood shed they caused was not dissimilar. They completely destroyed the Buddhist civilization of Gandhara, Taxila was looted, people massacred, monasteries burnt and demolished. The devastation was not just extensive it was total from which the Buddhism in Gandhara never recovered. The cities where famous monasteries were built were specially targeted obviously for the wealth they contained. After this destruction, centuries of desolation and dereliction the ruins were further obliterated by the earthquakes hitting the region regularly. The people did return and constructed their homes over the obliterated vestiges of their ancestors but Gandhara never regained its glory and lay buried till Taxila was discovered in late nineteenth century by the British archaeologists. It was then properly dug out in the early twentieth century by Sir John Marshall.[33] The evidence of large scale looting, killing, burning and absolute destruction by the White Huns has been specially noted by the archaeologists during excavations. There were no remains found of any wooden structures except charred remnants, skeletons were discovered with marks of violent injuries to cranium and other bones. Some valuables were discovered as if hurriedly hidden behind the false walls indicating that people were expecting the invasion and had a hope to return. Once the Huns completed the destruction of Gandhara and established themselves, they turned towards south and clashed with the Gupta dynasty in about 454 CE, when Kumara Gupta was killed but the Gupta rule survived only limited to a much reduced area.[34] In about 500 CE one of the descendants of White Huns, Toramana and then his son Mihirakula controlled Gandhara, Kashmir and all of the Panjab. Eventually their power declined that led to the establishment of a number of larger or smaller Rajputs city states, constantly fighting with each other. But they forced their way into the caste system as warriors and over a long period were assimilated mostly in agriculture. They can hardly claim to have patronised any form of art or learning or medicine, on the contrary they were undoubtedly the

---

[33] Marshall J. *Taxila* (3 volumes), Cambridge: Cambridge University Press, 1951.

[34] See note 31 above, pp. 66-70.

destroyers of what the Buddhists had created during the previous centuries. The decline of Buddhist medicine and surgery may also be attributed to this invasion. The historians have also produced evidence regarding the later Rajputs states were the remnants of the White Huns after their central power had declined.[35] Some of their clans inhabited in the region of Gandhara are known as Jats, Gujjars, Comboh and even Pathans were eventually settled mainly in agriculture in Panjab and present North West of present Pakistan.

The site at Taxila has been almost continuously excavated for about a century, yet new discoveries are made all the time and it seems lot more is still buried not only with in the boundaries of Taxila but more so at many other sites all over what was Gandhara. Many valuable discoveries of rock carvings are scattered in the inaccessible mountains, few have been discovered others are still waiting to be found.[36] From Kabul to Taxila wherever methodical archaeological excavations have been carried out, among the minor artefacts occasionally a medical item or even a proper surgical instrument has been identified. We learn from the Chinese travellers that this is also the area where many Buddhist monasteries were created in natural or artificially carved caves; these were inhabited by large number of monks. For a large population of monks and lay visiting pilgrims to these remote cave monasteries some kind of medical facilities must have been provided. When these sites are explored the medical artefacts are discovered.

The archaeologists of older school were more interested and found it exciting when huge stone sculptures, jewellery or coins were discovered while smaller pieces were always

---

[35] Smith VA. *The early history of India*, Oxford: The Clarendon Press, 1924, pp. 334-42.

[36] Jettmar K, Thewalt V. *Between Gandhara and the Silk Road, rock carvings along the Karakoram Highway*, 1987.

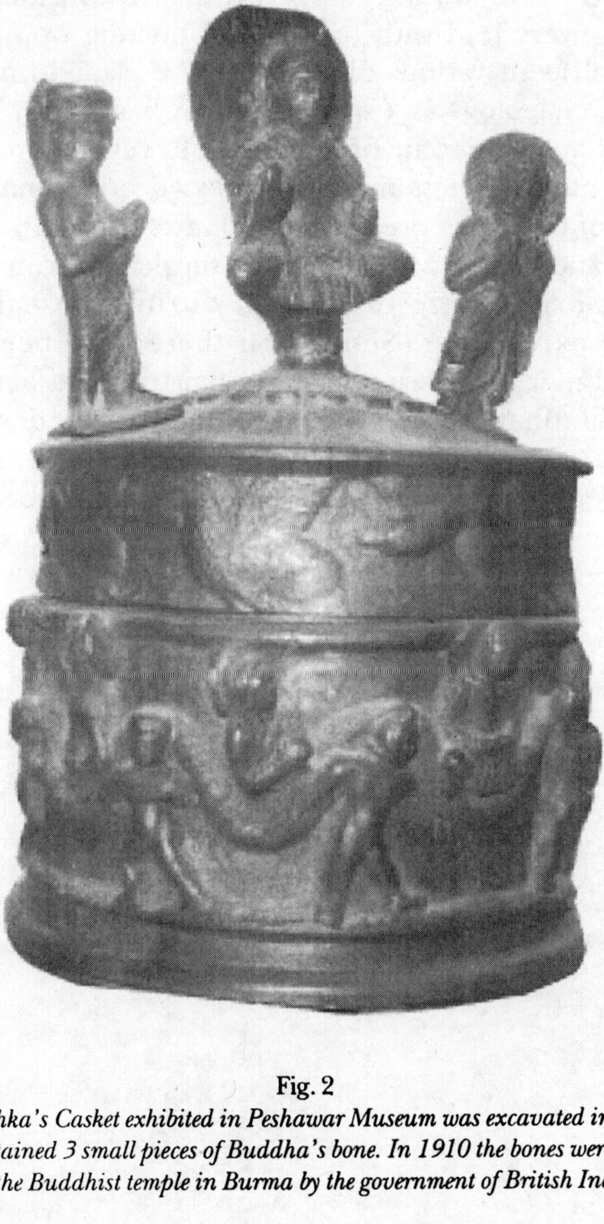

Fig. 2

Kanishka's Casket exhibited in Peshawar Museum was excavated in 1909, it contained 3 small pieces of Buddha's bone. In 1910 the bones were gifted to the Buddhist temple in Burma by the government of British India.

lumped under the heading of minor objects and not taken as seriously as big beautiful sculptures. The modern investigators fortunately have different emphasis and approach every find with open mind inviting opinions of the specialists in various disciplines. The establishment of medical archaeology as a special branch has greatly helped to identify and save some of the medically related finds. The fruits of this awareness may be witnessed occasionally and the news of newly discovered surgical artefacts often seen in the press and media. Majority of the surgical instruments of Buddhist origin were discovered during the early but extensive excavations. Since then there have been only occasional new discoveries of surgical instruments at various sites in Gandhara. Since the recently discovered surgical instruments from other sites have not been diligently studied and not yet been appraised by experts, these will be briefly discussed at the appropriate place during the discussion in the forthcoming pages.

2.
Archaeological sites of Taxila

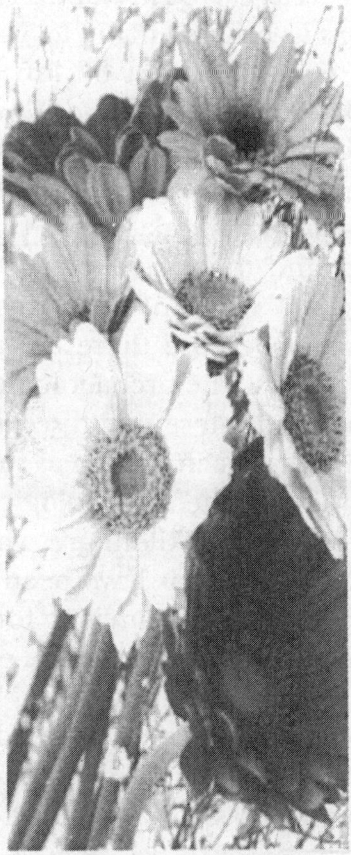

It has been pointed out in preceding pages that the city of Taxila is not mentioned by any name in the *Rig-Veda* but the post Vedic literature such as *Vayu Purana, Ramayana, Mahabharata* and nearly all the early Buddhist sacred texts it is mentioned by its Sanskrit name of *Takshasila.* This original Sanskrit name has been interpreted variously by different authors but most popular description that many historians agree is 'a city carved in stone'. This was Hellenised by the Greeks from its original name to Taxila. The modern city of Taxila is situated about 30 km from the capital Islamabad in Pakistan, while on the World map Taxila is positioned at 33.44 N and 72.49 E. Although Taxila was destroyed completely as mentioned in the above chronology, the people returned and populated the place over the ruins of their ancestors and today you may see villages next to excavations (Fig.3). Some of the sites have not been completely excavated because there are age old dwellings over them. Nevertheless the archaeological sites of Taxila the most important and interesting discoveries in the whole of subcontinent and has been graded as the World Heritage by the UNESCO (Fig.4). The archaeological sites are spread in a radius of well over ten kilometre where at numerous places intermittent excavations have been going on for the last 100 years or so and new ancient locations are often discovered revealing valuable artefacts. For a detailed story of the archaeology of Taxila the survey by Sir John Marshall in three volumes cited above is a must reading but for an up to date account Ahmad Hasan Danni's publication *Taxila* is a highly recommended essential account.[37] A comparative

[37] See note 11 above.

study of these two major works makes it clear how outlook may change once the new evidence came to light during subsequent excavations. In this respect the excavations carried out since 1968 are quite significant. This activity has revealed the habitation of late Neolithic period extending up to the period of 3000 BCE. At some places artefacts from third and second century BCE have also been recovered. The new discoveries pertaining to pre historic Gandhara are quite exciting for the archaeologists and historians but not yet fully assessed in publications.

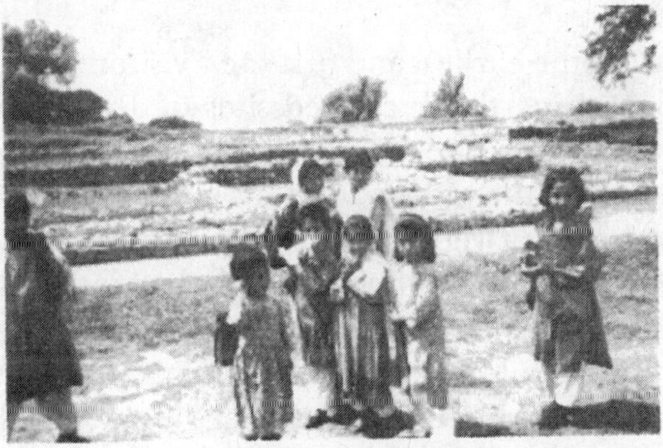

Fig. 3
School girls from their village walk through the ruins of ancient university on the way to school

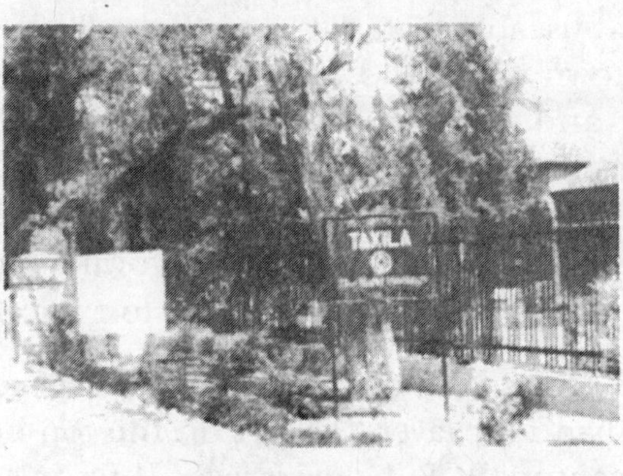

Fig. 4
The entrance to Taxila Museum

From general archaeological point of view the ancient ruins of Taxila are scattered in a huge area and it is acknowledged that much more is still hidden under the earth. Even a brief account of what is already exposed would be out side the scope of present discussion. But in order to complete the story a short introduction to those sites where surgical instruments and other related objects were discovered is also essential. Most important sites which are relevant to present discussion are listed below and briefly described in the next few paragraphs.

Bhir Mound

Bhir Mound is the earliest and first site a visitor will encounter when approaching the excavated sites of Taxila, only a few minutes walk from the Taxila train station. If travelling towards north by the old and famous Grand Trunk road the road sign directs a right turn to the archaeological sites, which are about 5 km after crossing the barrier at the railway crossing. The Taxila train station is on left, Bhir Mound site is on the right while the road ahead after a short distance leads to the Taxila Museum. The archaeological investigations at Bhir Mound did not reveal any regular pattern of a walled city, instead lot of broken stones were scattered around where the city wall should have been. It is just possible that damage by natural calamities was extensive; while it is also plausible that useable material from the wall was taken away to the new town which was sited not very far. On the same count no grand building of a temple, stupa, school or university was discovered intact at the Bhir Mound site. The streets are narrow that twist and turn in an irregular fashion. It is also possible that part of the ancient town is buried under the modern buildings and roads and is lost for good.

The archaeologists have discovered evidence that Bhir Mound site had four layers, layer I on the top belonged to the second century BCE, below it layer II fits in to about 3rd century or Mauryan period. The layer III has been allocated to the 4th century BCE and lowest layer IV dates back to 5th

century BCE. Although the archaeologists found it difficult to accurately demarcate depths of relevant layers, still such differentiation is important because it helps to place or assign a period to the artefacts discovered at various depths. The above classification was established on the evidence of excavations during early 20th century. New evidence as a result of digging carried out since 1968, throws light resulting in a different viewpoint. The deepest layers have revealed artefacts from the Neolithic period; this evidence puts the site at least 600 years back and renders Taxila one of those few cities that are continuously inhabited from Stone Age till today. On the evidence of the fresh excavations it is claimed by the investigators that the remains of a hall they have unearthed might be the remains of the palace where king of Taxila Ambhi entertained Alexander in 326 BCE. Further information on this discovery and the material unearthed is still under study. This is also a place that might reveal artefacts from Vedic period. For the keen visitors of today it must be emphasized that after excavations and studying the archaeology the site was again filled with rubble and what is now exposed and visible are the stones of the walls. Such an action was essential in order to protect the site from further ravages by the nature and man.

The deeper layers at Bhir Mound revealed some objects from the Achaemenian period, most importantly the coins that were found in large numbers fully corroborate with the historical accounts. Alexander was welcomed here and stayed a short period to replenish supplies for his army before the next important battle with Porus. Some other finds of luxury items include beads, jewellery of gold and silver and rings made of copper were also discovered during recent excavations. From layers or the stratum belonging to pre Mauryan and Mauryan period a number of copper objects and iron tools were discovered. Among these were two surgical instruments of copper and suturing needles made of iron.

Sirkap

It has been mentioned earlier that the foundation of a new city Sirkap in Taxila was laid in about middle of the second century BCE. It was designed on a typical Greek grid pattern, which can be seen on the city plan prepared after the excavation of the whole city; the streets are straight crossing each other at right angle. The city was protected by a strong wall on all sides. This city during first three centuries changed hands from Bactrian Greeks, Sakas, Parthians, and the Kushans. In second century CE it was replaced by the third new city called Sirsukh founded by the third Kushan king Kanishka. Sirkap occupies the largest area among all archaeological sites that have been brought to light since the first excavations were carried out. Although it was primarily a Buddhist town yet many other religious temples have been discovered, which makes it a cosmopolitan city where all were free to practice what ever faith they prefer. In the wide main street of Sirkap you may see the remains of a number of Buddhist Stupa, Zoroastrian, Jain and Hindu temples. A broad-based progressive and prosperous nature of this city can also be judged by the number of shops that existed in the main street. In one such shop a large stone has been recognized as the work shop of a jeweller, where along with ornaments other delicate objects would also be made (Fig.5).

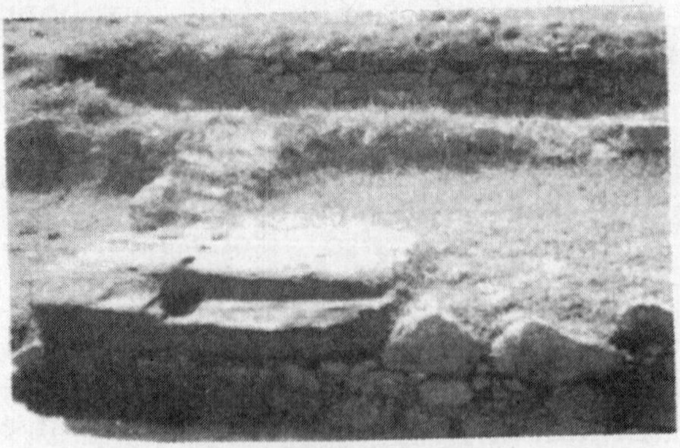

Fig. 5

A jeweller's workshop at Sirkap showing the stone used in the trade

A large majority of art pieces that are exhibited under the label of Gandhara sculptures not only in Taxila museum but many other museums all over the World were excavated from this site. The sheer number and variety of trade items discovered here further points to a liberal nature of Sirkap where different people were free to conduct their business. In such a complex but prosperous society medical and surgical skills must be needed and in demand, accordingly the practitioners of medicine and surgery must be skilful in their profession. Such a view is fully corroborated by the discovery of surgical instruments and pharmaceutical objects that were discovered in Sirkap. The dynamism of this city can also be judged from the number of sculptures of great splendour that have filled the museums all over the World and private collections.

There are two historical traditions which recount the interest of the kings ruling in Sirkap who demonstrated an eager interest in other religions and also in philosophical discourses. According to an apocryphal tradition the Apostle Thomas visited Taxila and had a dialogue with Gonophores king at Sirkap in about 40 CE.[38] Among the ruins of Sirkap there is a platform where even today local Christian community assembles once a year to celebrate the visit of Apostle Thomas.

According to another tradition shortly after the visit of Apostle Thomas the Roman philosopher Apollonius of Tania also visited Taxila and engaged in the discussion with Gonophores in his capital Sirkap.[39] These exchanges no doubt show that Taxila was a melting pot where apart from religion, secular sciences such as arts, philosophy, medicine and other disciplines were cultivated and taught in various

---

[38] Farquhar JN. 'The Apostle Thomas in North India, *John Rylands Library Bulletin* 1927, pp. 20-50. Also see Medlycott AE. *India and the Apostle Thomas, an inquiry with a critical analysis of the Acta Thomae,* London: David Nutt, 1905.

[39] Phillimore JS. tr., *Philostratus in honour of Appollonius of Tania,* Oxford: 1912.

schools, some were elevated to the same level what we regard as a present day university.

A royal residence or a Palace was discovered at the most southern end of Sirkap while further higher up overlooking the city the archaeologists discovered ruins of another grand building recognized as *Mahal* (Royal residence). This much larger site within Sirkap has been dated to be from early Kushan period or first century CE. A number of luxury items like jewellery, silver plates and coins were discovered during excavations. Apart from many objects a decapitator was also unearthed from this site. Sir John Marshall has also speculated that the ruins of this building indicate extensive damage as a result of massive earthquake, which hit Taxila in the first or second decade of CE.

The Dharmarajika Stupa

The Dharmarajika Stupa is another important historical site situated about 5 kilometres south east of the museum; it is approached by a path involving crossing the old rivulet Tamara over the stepping stones. Its name suggests it was first built by Ashoka but probably altered and rebuilt many times since. On two counts it is the largest and most sacred place discovered any where in Gandhara. First it was built by Ashoka and secondly it housed the most sacred relic. The site is dotted with many smaller stupas all around the main great central stupa of Dharmarajika. The great stupa was surrounded by a wide platform which was paved with unique glass tiles, some of these are exhibited in the museum. The glass was never manufactured in Gandhara; these square tiles must have been imported from Roman Empire. The platform was used for circumvention by the monks and pilgrims who came to perform their religious rites. According to Sir John Marshall who was the first to carry out excavations, the great stupa was broken in by robbers probably some time in the previous century in search of valuables. The relic of Buddha's bone was discovered not in the great stupa but in a smaller stupa nearer the steps of the great stupa. In a golden reliquary that was placed inside another casket along with a ruby there was a small piece of bone. This was deposited by Ashoka when he distributed Buddha's bones to different sacred places in his kingdom. After its discovery this incredibly sacred relic was handed over as a present to the Buddhists of Ceylon (Sri Lanka) in 1917. The decision to gift it to the then Ceylon was made by the then British Indian government in return for political advantages. The relic is now installed in the World famous Temple of the Tooth at Kandy in Sri Lanka.[40]

The site of Dharmarajika is also significant owing to the discovery of at least one substantial surgical instrument that will be discussed later. In addition its long monastic connection also associate it with medical and surgical practice because surgery in particular was the vacation of the monks living in monasteries where people visited in huge numbers seeking spiritual guidance and treatment as well.

Sirsukh

When Kushan took the control of Gandhara they kept Sirkap as their capital for two generations, it was the third king Kanishka who decided to build a new city and move his headquarters from Sirkap to the new city. Why such decision was made has been a matter of many speculations. In the opinion of Sir John Marshall the old Greek city Sirkap 'had been visited by a deadly plague which whipped out half the inhabitants, and that only two or three decade earlier it had been laid in ruins by a devastating earthquake'.[41] But we are not sure if this is pure assumption because Sir John Marshall has not offered any convincing evidence to verify it. It seems futile to build a new capital just a short walking distance from the plague infested old city because it will not offer any protection. Moreover the old city was not abandoned entirely while its buildings remained intact and the stones

---

[40] See note 33 above, vol. 1, p. 242.

[41] See note 33 above, vol. 1, p. 217.

were not used to build the new Sirsukh. A simple and more logical explanation might be that Sirkap was over populated and since geographical restrictions it cannot be expanded any further, a satellite town only a short distance away was raised by the wish of a really powerful emperor probably for his elite aristocracy. It was surrounded by a protection wall which had almost disappeared and only a trace of the outer wall was discovered when a series of trenches were dug at different locations. Only limited archaeological excavations have been carried out at Sirsukh site due to village life within its boundaries. At this site probably great many surprise discoveries are waiting for the future archaeologists. Among some of the usual finds discovered from limited pits dug at less intruding places there were coins, bone and ivory, beads, copper objects, shell jewellery, pottery and stone decorations. Sirsukh has the potential to yield surgical instruments or other related items due to strong medical history during the reign of Kanishka. If Caraka ever practised medicine it must be at this place.

Mohra Moradu

Mohra Moradu is the ancient name and village with this name still exists about 1.5 kilometres in south-easterly direction of Sirkap. Away from the village and higher up on the hill there is a Buddhist monastery and a substantial stupa, the stupa and the village both carry the same name (Fig.6). The site must have been selected by the Buddhists builders for its natural picturesque splendour, where they constructed an ideal place for meditation in a small basin surrounded by green hills. The place really inspires spirituality. A path after crossing a stream ascends to the site away from the village; as you walk on the path on right side there is a deep cave that was filled with water fed from the stream, which is now almost dried up but must be the source of water for the monastery in its hey-days. Today we see modern water channel carrying water from a dam many miles upstream running under a new bridge before disappearing into a tunnel under the hill not far from the

Stupa. When the stupa was first discovered it was found to be exceptionally well decorated, the walls all around were covered with highly decorative figures of Buddha and Bodhisattvas of extraordinary elegance. Mohra Moradu is the site which yielded the most interesting objects along with the finest life-size sculpture of Gandhara art ever discovered in the form of Bodhisattva Maitreya. The stupa at Mohra Moradu is now recognized to be the Kunala Stupa depicted in the legend of Ashoka's son Kunala who was blinded after his step mother treacherously accused him for making advance to her. When his eye sight was miraculously restored the stupa became a place of pilgrimage for those seeking cure for eye ailments. Although for a long time another stupa situated at the southern side of Sirkap over a hill had been mistakenly associated where this miracle happened. The record now has been set right after accurate description of this site that the Chinese traveller Hsuan Tsang had recorded in his travels.[42] An elevated spiritual value of this site because of association with the miracle involving Ashoka's son is indicative why it acquired the amazing sacred aura during the Buddhist period.

The details of the monastery of Mohra Moradu described by Hsuan Tsang clearly identifies this site with a place where large number of Buddhist monks were in residence and the place attracted pilgrims who came for spiritual guidance as well as cures for the physical diseases. The size of this monastery was big enough where the monks would have performed the healing, teach and train the young apprentices and other related activities such as processing of medicines would be carried out. One historian has summarized such activities in the Buddhist monasteries of Taxila and their status as centre of excellence in the following words.[43]

---

[42] See note 11 above, p.141.

[43] Zysk KG. *Asceticism and healing in ancient India,* Oxford: Oxford University Press, 1991, p. 47.

Taxila was therefore an excellent venue for the establishment of a symbolic relationship between medical education and Buddhist monasticism.

The tradition of nursing the ill and treating the ailing *bhiksus* living in the monasteries was laid by the Buddha himself during his life time. From this tradition the Buddhists Monks considered it their religious duty to provide the medical care to the resident monks and extended their charity to the pilgrims as well who were in need for such help. Naturally the surgical treatments must also be part of the comprehensive medical service which was provided with in the monasteries. It was this back ground that most Buddhist monasteries became the centre where people will go to seek medical cure. The monastery of Mohra Moradu during the peak of Buddhist period acquired a kind of approbation as a popular place of pilgrimage where cure particularly of the diseases of the eye was available and the legend carried on, attracting pilgrims who for centuries came to worship, seek spiritual guidance and also anticipated cure for eye ailments because they strongly believed in the miracle of Kunala.

The mystical and spiritual folklore about this place is still alive, even today the place is visited by many and it is now known as *PanjpOir* or the dwelling of five saints.

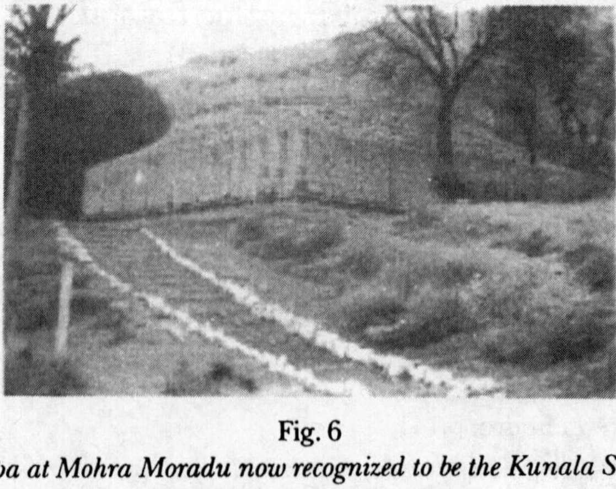

Fig. 6

Stupa at Mohra Moradu now recognized to be the Kunala Stupa on the evidence of Hsuan Tsang.

3.
The Taxila School

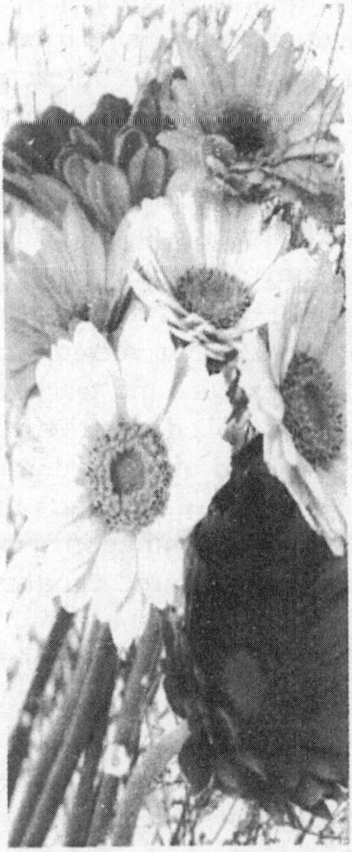

All those who have written history of ancient education in India consistently agree that Taxila was a centre of excellence for the teaching of all disciplines. The post Vedic Sanskrit literature and ancient Buddhist sacred books have described Taxila the capital of Gandhara and a centre of learning or a kind of intellectual centre equivalent to present day university town. The fame of great scholars and specialist teachers of Taxila attracted students from far and wide. The historians have mentioned names of teachers of philosophy, theology, grammar, astrology, mathematicians, medicine and surgery. The students came at a young age from royal or noble families as well as common youngsters who wanted to pursue the path of learning. On the evidence of these texts it seems that for many centuries a system or tradition was evolved where the parents of well off students paid fee to the teacher but poorer students served the teacher in return for his teaching.[44] In practice the teacher's family adopted the young students and looked after them till they completed the education. The period of medical graduation has been described to be seven years, at the end of which the student has to under go a final examination. Few of the legendry teachers from Taxila had acquired a godly status, in Buddhist stipulations they had received the enlightenment but they had decided to live and serve the people on the earth. On the other hand in Taxila there were others who never attained sainthood still achieved historical fame due to their secular contributions to medicine or other sciences. Few of these are known to history others shall always remain anonymous.

[44] See note 10 above, pp. 477-91.

For a moment if we just restrict ourselves to surgery then we find that despite the remoteness of the period and obliteration of the evidence due to the elapse of long period, few archaeological objects in the form of surgical implements that have been unearthed in Taxila throw intriguing light on the remarkable efforts of those who must have used these objects to pe. form surgical procedures. The historical worth of these objects is not because these are the only surgical artefacts discovered but more so in the facts that they represent the skills in metallurgy, designing and manufacturing of the artisans of Gandhara. They also represent the expertise of surgeons who used then and off course no doubt they also reflect the suffering of patients who endured the pain and sufferings. If we keep in mind their social impact then the historical backdrop of Taxila being a centre of excellence for medical teaching emerges far greater than it has been painted by the historians. Taxila appears to be the only place out side Geek and Roman lands where surgical instruments have been excavated by the archaeologists. This distinction is owing to the fact that the surgical instruments excavated in Taxila are comparable with the Greek and Roman instruments and no where else in the World similar objects have been discovered.

At this stage it is proper to discuss some legendary persons or semi historical people from Taxila who were associated with medicine and surgery and some others who were linked with secular sciences. The first two mentioned in the following pages must have acted as surgeons during their career as indicated by the sketches recorded in various sources of their historical deeds. We should not expect that there were specialist surgeons performing surgical procedures only; they were teachers of medicine or came to Taxila to learn medicine and during their professional life offered surgical treatments if required or operate when faced with no alternative to surgical intervention. After all surgery has always been a risky business with high mortality and all through the ages was employed only when there was absolutely no other option. It is amazing reality that despite high risks and likelihood of awful publicity in likely circumstance of loosing the patient, the bravery of surgeons was such that never diminished their spirits.

There is hardly any biographical information about the individuals, some names are known only because they have left texts of enduring eminence. Some other personalities from Taxila will be included in discussion when the medical texts they are associated with will be discussed at a later stage. There are few other names who were not directly involved in medicine but their stature is such that any discussion on Taxila without them will be meaningless.

Atreya

One legendary medical teacher who taught in Taxila was Atreya; his name indicates that he belonged to the cast of Atri mentioned in the earliest texts as scholars and teachers. Atreya is a celebrated towering figure who achieved a saintly eminence and revered by all later authors. The legends surrounding him tell us that he received the medical knowledge directly from the gods and was accorded the responsibility to pass it on through his pupils for the benefit of humanity. The existence of legendary Atreya is difficult to pinpoint on historical time line. But if any real person ever walked and taught in Taxila by the name of Atreya it must be in remote past. There are plentiful references to Atreya in the Buddhists sources. In *Mahavagga,* which is the second book of the most sacred Buddhist text *The Vinaya Pitaka,* was probably compiled around second or third century CE. It mentions Atreya many times as the teacher residing in Taxila who also taught medicine to Jivaka (see below). At the same time the non-Buddhist Sanskrit texts also portray him the great teacher who taught medicine and surgery in Taxila.[45] These sources go to the extent to bestow

[45] Filliozat J. *The classical doctrine of Indian medicine,* Channa DR, tr., Delhi: Munshiram Manoharlal Oriental Booksellers and Publishers, 1964.

the ultimate honour to Atreya as the originator of Ayurvedic medicine, who taught and trained six pupils, Agnivesa, Bhela, Harita, Jatukarna, Parasara, and Ksirrapani. His six pupils in turn took his teaching far and wide by recording and compiling his teachings once they completed their education and moved to their respective abodes. Most of their works have been lost in the sand of time but three texts by first three pupils named above are generally believed to be extant. Among these three one text that is associated with Agnivesa being the primary author is the famous *Caraka Samhita*. While a single copy of *Bhela Samhita* is claimed to be discovered in incomplete, damaged or corrupt form. The third known as *Harita Samhita* remains elusive and obscure. We are also told that *Bhela Samhita* in some form was available to the authors of the *Bower manuscript* because at least three formulae from this have been quoted in the *Bower manuscript.*

However the name of Jivaka is not included among those six pupils mentioned above, his name only comes into picture as the pupil of Atreya in Taxila primarily from the Buddhist texts.

The historical Atreya is also mentioned by almost all the medical historians of Indian medicine, in fact the earliest Indian medicine or Ayurveda cannot be set in to historical motion without Atreya because most believe he was the interface between gods and human beings. Every chapter of *Caraka Samhita* begins with an avowal, 'thus spake the worshipful Atreya', and ends with the words, 'thus spake worshipful Punarvasu'. Punarvasu Atreya might be an honorific or full name of the person normally referred as Atreya. The controversy as regard to this name has been end less in Indian literature; some have argued that Punarvasu Atreya is altogether different person belonging to the South. This might be due to the traditional un-ending North-South rivalry perceptible from ancient, medieval and even in modern literature.

A large majority of writers if not all agree that Atreya was the most famous medical professor at the time when Taxila was at its zenith offering all kind of medical learning to his followers. Further more the historians also concur that Atreya's period was about the time of Buddha or not long before the birth of Buddha. It would be reasonable assumption that historical Atreya lived about the time of Achaemenian conquest or middle of 6th century BCE. This analysis best fits with the concept recorded in Buddhist sacred books that Atreya was the foremost teacher in Taxila who trained Jivaka for seven years before Jivaka was ready and travelled to serve as Buddha's personal doctor. This sketch of historical events has been drawn and recorded by many authorities.[46] Yet more proof of historical Atreya has been put forward by others from the existence of a manuscript which is known as *Atreya Samhita* in British Library catalogue number 2640 consisting of 164 folios. There is no translation or editorial work ever been carried out on this apparently mysterious document about which little is known including its period, the circumstances of its discovery and even its authenticity?

From the above scrutiny of historical events a few facts come out very clearly to us. We know that Gandhara was the first station on the road of Aryan migration and gradually transformed into a region of progress and prosperity. At the same time the post-Vedic Sanskrit literature similarly mentions Takshasila the capital of Gandhara and also became a great place of learning. It is no surprise that Taxila gradually became a specialised centre of teaching where medicine was taught in an organised fashion. It was here that the Ayurvedic Medicine was evolved as a scientific and rational system and Atreya was the earliest teacher. Atreya's teaching was first spread far and wide by his pupils and later by those who came to Taxila to learn and then took the knowledge with them to practise in far away places. The

[46] See note 27 above, p. xviii.

legend of Atreya is strongly associated with Taxila. But it is unfortunate that tradition of recording accurate historical chronology was not established and we can only rely on the fragmented information from limited sources available.

Jivaka

Jivaka is one of the most revered personalities because he was the personal doctor to no less than the Buddha himself and also a distinguished hero in numerous Jataka or stories recorded in Buddhist sacred books.[47] His legendry gallant life begins at his birth when he was left on a rubbish heap by his mother who was a courtesan and had no use for a boy. He was rescued by the orders of the prince Abhaya or son of King Bimbisara. Another legend goes that he was illegitimate son of prince Abhaya who adopted him. While others tell he was illegitimate son of King Bimbisara and brother of Abhaya. Despite all the disadvantages surrounded his birth Jivaka was brought up in the Royal household and at a very young age he was sent to Taxila to study medicine under the great teacher Atreya. Here he learnt medicine and at the end of the course that took seven years he was subjected to the final test of his abilities. He was given a horse and a spade and told to go around the hills and valleys of Taxila and bring to his teacher those plants that have no medicinal value. After the prescribed time of wanderings Jivaka returned to the teacher empty handed and passed the test with flying colours. Once he acquired his laurels he started the long journey to his home where his fate was destined to look after Lord Buddha himself and also heal others. There must be nearly one hundred stories in Buddhist sacred books about Jivaka's practise of medicine and surgery among masses and performing miraculous surgical feats. At times he was awarded rich rewards by the royalties or other rich people

[17] Fausbill V, *The Jatakas: together with its commentary, being tales of anterior birth of Gotama Buddha,* 7 volumes, Rhys Davis TW, tr., London: Trübner and Co, 1877-97. Also see Oldenberg H. *Sacred books of the East: Mahavagga,* Rhys Davis TW, tr., Oxford: Clarendon Press, 1882.

for successfully treating them or their loved ones. Jivaka is also known as Jivaka Kumarabhacca, which probably is an honour to describe him a children doctor because, traditions also record he had cured a child by performing an abdominal operation when the child developed life threatening internal condition. Another view put forward by some others is that there were two people with this name; one Vrdha Jivaka was a specialist in the diseases of children though his period remains unknown. The other named Jivaka was a surgeon who lived during the time of Buddha.[48] The time of Jivaka the surgeon is also close to what some propose and believe to be the time of the author of *Susruta Samhita.* It may not be preposterous to suggest that Jivaka seems to have all the qualifications and is a deserving candidate who might be considered as the rightful author of *Susruta Samhita.* After all he is the only one who repeatedly appears in most ancient texts as a surgeon. In Allahabad Museum the Terracotta showing a dissected abdomen, illustrated and highlighted below might have been sculpted to celebrate the surgical feats of Jivaka as surgeon.

In another story when Buddha's' foot was injured from the rock thrown at him by Devadatta it was Jivaka who cleaned the wound and applied the medicated bandage to the foot and advised rest. It is further recorded that after observing that the Buddhist monks living in the Monasteries were pale and looked sickly Jivaka persuaded Buddha to include regular exercise in the routines within the monastic life. The exemplary hardiness generally observed among the Buddhist monks might be due to Jivaka's fore thought on energetic healthy living.

Another story tells when Jivaka had to administer an unpleasant medication to Buddha; he prepared the medication and sprinkled it over three lotus flowers. These

---

[48] Mitra J. *A critical appraisal of Ayurvedic material in Buddhist literature: With special reference to Tripitaka,* Varanasi: Jyotirlok Prakashan, 1985, p. 329.

flowers were then given to Buddha who after smelling the flowers had the desired effect of the medicine that he had inhaled by smelling the lotus flowers. The story offers an insight that the concept of administering medication by inhalation was known in the time of Jivaka. The administration of medicines by inhalation has been reported by many later Buddhist medical and religious texts.

Although Jivaka has no historical authentication, a short comment recorded by Rudolf Hoernle and quoted below is worthy of taking note.[49]

Jivaka is a historical or semi historical personage.

It is difficult to figure out what to make out by a semi historical figure as recorded by the eminent historian. However the stories of Jivaka whether legendary or semi historical do depict him as a hard working medical practitioner who also performed valiant surgery whenever faced with the situation and gave his best to his patients that included godly persons, royalties, rich as well as poor. His life story of achieving a high position in his vocation despite thrown on rubbish heap after his birth no doubt sets a brilliant example, especially in the atmosphere of strict cast distinctions. The stories tell us that in his entire carrier he always showed readiness to help those who ever called upon him. The moral from his stories must have made profound impact and influenced many good Buddhists who followed in his foot steps finding contentment or enlightenment by serving the fellow beings with their surgical skills.

Jivaka the semi historical personality, who learned medicine in Taxila, became a personal physician to Buddha and the only named surgeon during a long period in history seems to have not left any text about his work or teachings.

---

[19] Hoernle AFR. *The Bower Manuscript: facsimile leaves, Nagari transcript, Romanised transliteration and English translation with notes,* Calcutta: Superintendent Government Printing, 1893-1912, p. lxii.

The only witnesses of his therapeutic legacy are the two prescriptions associated with his name that have been cited in the *Bower Manuscript.* One of the two formulae attributed to Jivaka is for the treatment of emesis and the other is to relive the spasm of the chest.[50] How the authors of the *Bower Manuscript* stumbled over these two prescriptions will always remain an enigma of history.

It is now imperative that after discussing the two most famous medical men, who were associated with Taxila, a brief mention is also made of others who did not make into the history books as medical men but their contributions in other areas of academic endeavours cannot be ignored even if we are primarily discussing the history of medical. Although it is also true that in ancient times learned people always had some knowledge of medicine and especially of plants that had properties of curing. The inclusion and brief mention of these most important figures also supports the status of Taxila as the centre of all kinds of learning during ancient times.

Panini

The most important personality in this respect mentioned above was no doubt of Panini and who would be better than him to commence this discussion. Irrespective of the fact that Panini was the greatest grammarian and primarily not a medical person even then no account on history of Gandhara or Taxila can be complete without including the name of Panini. If there is any one who can stand equal to the philosophers, mathematicians and other learned names from the classical Greek period then it is Panini. Panini compiled 4000 rules of grammar in his text based on highly technical and complex system comparable to the modern computer codes. It is surprising that from ancient times till now we can see virtually hundreds of texts critically evaluating his work but little is known or written about the man himself.

[50] See note 49 above, pp.178-80.

When one tries to explore Panini's personality only scant fragmented biographical information can be extracted from a number of surveys and texts on history of Sanskrit literature. To begin with the usual problem is encountered; the chroniclers for a long time have been engaged into the controversy regarding his time. He has been dated from 4th to 7th century BCE but it is finally accepted on the evidence derived from his own writing that Panini flourished during early to mid fourth century BCE.[51] He was born in a place that was known as Salatura or Shalatura on the right bank of the river Indus in the district of Attock (colonial name Campbellpur) in Pakistan. The place was not very far from Taxila. His name was first found on a copper plate of 7th century CE as Salaturiya, meaning one who was born in Salatura. He was also known as son of Daksi after his mother. His younger brother Pingala was famous for his scholarship in mathematics (see below). Hsuan Tsang tells us that during his travels when he visited Salatura he was told about Panini and that his statue existed at his birth place. Panini is also one of the few early secular authors who have mentioned Takshasila or Taxila in his gigantic work where he himself was a teacher. Winternitz referring an ancient Sanskrit text tells us that Panini was killed by a lion.[52]

Although Panini exclusively deals with grammar, in his text we find references to almost all aspects of life of his time. There is no detailed discussion on medicine at all in his writing except a brief mention of few diseases only in passing to illustrate points of grammar by citing examples. Such references to diseases and treatments only occur infrequently in different *sutras* in his famous text. As an example a leper is defined while explaining the function of an affix that describes a person suffering from leprosy. At

[51] Cardona G. 'Panini - a survey of research', in Winter W., ed., *Trends in Linguistics. State- of-the-art-report 6,* Paris: Mouton, 1976, pp. 260-68.

[52] Winternitz M. *History of Indian literature,* Jha S, tr., Delhi: Motilal Banarsidass, 1967, pp. 420-30.

another place vomiting, diarrhoea, itch-scab and head ache are mentioned not in medical context but to demonstrate the use of an affix.[53] Although as mentioned above an ephemeral interest in medicine was always part of learning among the ancient intellectuals and polymaths and Panini must had such interest.

The singular gift and unique contribution of this most famous son of Gandhara was to set the laws of Sanskrit grammar in his *Astadhyayi,* meaning eight books or chapters. In a text where rules of grammar are laid it is not expected that there would be discussion on medicine.[54] Few names of medical conditions that Panini has recorded as examples and have been described above are only to make a point how words are formed with the rules of grammar. In an indirect way brief reference of few diseases Panini has alluded to further validate presence of well established and systematic medicine and medical teaching in Taxila where Panini was also a teacher. This view has been put forwards by the authors of *History of Indian literature* in these words.[55]

> That Indian medicine had in Panini's time already attained a certain degree of cultivation appears from the names of certain diseases specified by him.

In recent years Panini was honoured on a postal stamp issued in 2004 in India (Fig.7). The image on the stamp has been designed to show and implies that Panini is writing in Kharoshthi characters.

---

[53] Vasu SC. ed. and tr., *The Ashtadhyayi of Panini,* Delhi: Motilal Banarsidass, Reprint 1997, vol.1, p. 522 and vol. 2, p. 941.

[54] MacDonnell AA. *A history of Sanskrit literature,* London: W. Heinemann, 1900.

[55] Weber A, Mann J, Zacharia T. trs., *The history of Indian literature,* London: Kegan Paul, Trench, Trübner, 1892, pp. 265-71.

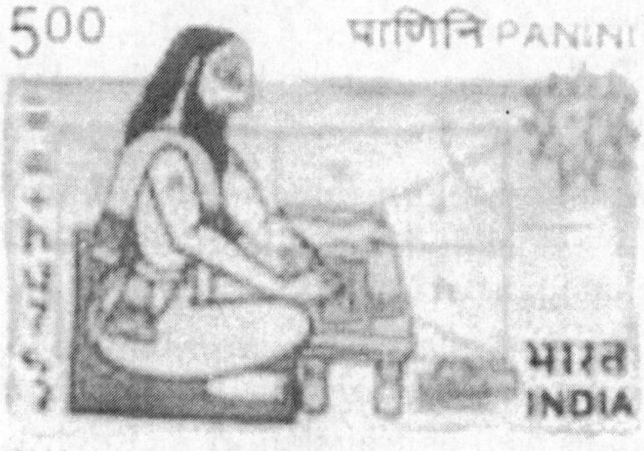

Fig. 7

Stamp issued by Indian Post in 2004 to honour Panini

Herewith it will be sufficient to mention only briefly about few others who were not medical men but their association with Taxila can be historically verified from different reliable sources reinforcing the standing of Taxila as a centre of learning.

Pingala

Mother Daksi must be a proud woman who gave birth to Panini the grammarian and his younger brother Pingala the mathematician. The fundamental contributions of the two brothers in grammar and mathematics are enough to make Gandhara proud of her two great sons. Pingala must be the first theorist who described the basic components of musical notes on mathematical grounds. His work *Chandas Sastra* though has not survived but glimpses of this earliest musical theory have emerged from the commentaries of later writers. In this unique work Pingala seems to touch the most important mathematical theories that during later period emerged as Binomial Theorem and even the Fibonacci Numbers. Although in this early work Pingala had meant to write a treatise on Prosody and how the syllabic combinations can be put together in poetical or musical expressions. His description of short and long syllables in metric construction is also considered first example of binary system in mathematics.

Vyadi

The little known but important philosopher Vyadi was been associated with Taxila where he flourished about 400 BCE, though not much biographical information is available about Vyadi. But his associated with the Taxila School has been recorded by reliable historians. His scholarly work has survived mainly through Patanjali and a number of manuscripts of his philosophical works are now available under the heading of *Paribhasavrtti* as well as translation in English by modern writers.[56]

Patanjali

Patanjali flourished during second century BCE or little later, he is known to have written a tom on Sanskrit grammar expounding on the Panini's grammar. His name is also associated with the first text on Yoga but not accepted uniformly by all.

Kautilya or Canakya

Kautilya or Canakya or Chanakya are different names of the same person, who also attended the school of Taxila and remained a trusted minister during the reign of first two Mauryan emperors dying at an advance age. According to *Encyclopaedia Britannica* he was a Zoroastrian and also had extensive medical knowledge. It is true that there was Zoroastrian population in Taxila after the Achaemenian conquest of Gandhara, which can be archaeologically confirmed by the remains of a Zoroastrian temple that was discovered in Taxila. The strength of Mauryan Empire was mostly due to his intelligent council. He wrote *Arthasastra* in Taxila and it is also possible that the first Mauryan Emperor Chandragupta was his student in Taxila during his young age.[57] Although it is a treatise on government but it also

---

[56] Cardona G. 'A new edition of Vyadi's *Paribhasavrtti*', *Journal of the American Oriental Society*, Vol.118:1998.

[57] Dani AH. 'Pre-Muslim period', in Qureshi IH, ed., *A short history of Pakistan*, Book I, Karachi: Karachi University Press, 1992.

contains many references to medicine. Even though there are only scanty references to medical treatments in Kautilya's writing, yet these are of interest when compared with the medical compendiums of Caraka and Susruta or the Greek medical texts of the contemporary period of Herophilus and Erasistratus. From these glimpses we may surmise the state of medicine around the time of Mauryan Empire. This may be illustrated from the story which recounts that Kautilya used to feed King Chandragupta some kind of poison in his food in order to build up his resistance against poisoning by an enemy. Once the queen who was pregnant shared the food and died. Kautilya immediately performed a caesarean section and saved the child who succeeded as King Bindusara to the Mauryan Empire. At another place where preparation of invasion of the enemy territory is discussed Kautilya gives sound advice to the kings with regard to fulfilling the medical needs and heartening the army.[58]

> Physicians with surgical instruments (*sastra*) medicines, remedial oils and cloth in their hands; and women with prepared food and beverages should stand behind, uttering encouraging words to fighting men.

After this brilliant spark in the *Arthasastra* whole of the book XIV titled 'Secret Means' and extended over many chapters is full of prescriptions containing most diabolical ingredients and conjurations to cast injury and death spells on adversaries. A sample of this may be gleaned in the following example.

> The smoke caused by burning the skin of a snake, the dung of a cow and horse, and the head of blind snake causes blindness.

Parts of the animals and of various plants have been mentioned profusely to be used both in the magical potions

---

[58] Kautilya, *Arthasastra,* Shamasastry R, tr., Bangalore: Government Press, 1915, pp. 495-54.

as well as in medicines. But in this chapter these are not employed to correct the imbalances or to restore the equilibrium of the five elements as taught in the Ayurvedic empirical system, but to cast spells, mostly to cause harm to enemies. Kautilya's *Arthasastra* being earlier than the two revised treatises of *Caraka Samhita* and *Susruta Samhita* offers us an insight into what might be the medical practice before the Ayurveda was established on rational foundation. This process was first established by the Buddhists in Gandhara. Similar information may also be interpreted from some of the other texts belonging to a period before the word Ayurveda was introduced in the medical literature.

4.
Evidence of surgery from sculptures

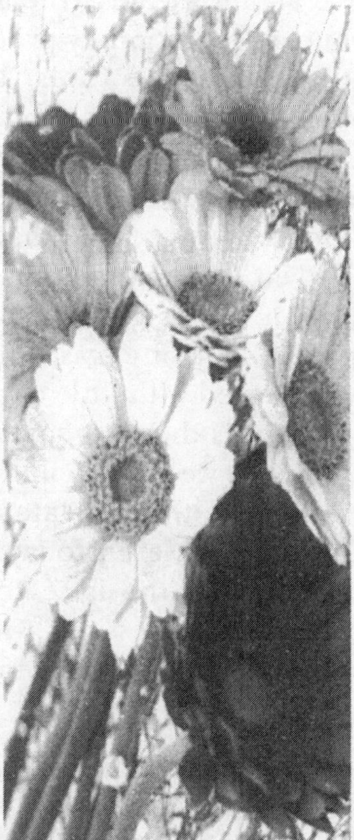

Almost all ancient civilizations have left iconic images or writings representing their cultural traditions, such records may be seen today in the form of sculptures or epigraphy. The imagery reflecting many aspects of life etched on stone or written on stone is found in abundance in all museums. In other words stone happen to be the only medium that has always played an important role in recording the achievements of human evolutionary process from the time man designed the first stone tools. If the Egyptians, Harappan, Mesopotamians, Greeks, Romans, Chinese and Indians had not left records of their society on endurable medium of stone our understanding of the World history would have been poorer. We are told that God also handed over to Moses the Ten Commandments carved on stone. The human emulation of this godly act and engraving his deeds of glorification on stone was worth all the efforts because these have survived with little damage from ravages of time. In many instances the history written or carved on stone is the only evidence we have to understand the events and interpret the past. Although later in history other materials were also used but even today whenever human deification is celebrated stone is selected as preferred medium. The proverbial expression 'written on stone' is justifiably used in most languages meaning some thing that is indestructible.

When it comes to illustrate the human achievements in medicine and surgery it is disappointing that the epigraphy and sculptures representing medical themes are not only scanty but we may say almost non existent, a reality uniformly found among all the civilizations. As an example when we look for surgery related epigraphical evidence it is minuscule as compared to the depiction of other human activity. There is probably one Egyptian carving representing circumcision that has been cited above and only a few more from Greek and Roman periods in the form of busts of well known people and only an hand full more representing surgical instruments.

Some writers of Indian medical history have looked and presented the evidence of surgery from the ancient sculptures and have presented such material as unequivocal evidence in support of surgery during the remote past of Indian history. This indirect kind of evidence traditionally has always found its place in the beginning of historical writings to which historiographers generally do not take seriously. In case of surgery it is certainly considered only a sketchy support for the practice of any serious surgery. One publication from 1938 referred two carvings where the story of King Sivi is illustrated, putting up the argument that this is substantial evidence that the surgery was widely practiced in ancient India.[59] The same line of reasoning has been repeated and talked about by others with or without the reference to the original paper. Let us find the background details and reality of these sculptures and what their purpose was in the minds of those who executed them and what we can learn today from these art objects.

The story of King Sivi or Sibi may be seen recorded in two different versions. One version is in *Mahabharata,* where King Sivi was audaciously put to test by gods Agni and Indra; one of them turned into a dove and the other into a hawk. The dove chased by the hawk takes refuge under the throne of King Sivi and begged the king her life must be saved, while the hawk flew in to demand his hard earned fair meal. The king offers better and bigger meals but the hawk would only accept the dove. At last King Sivi offers his own flesh

---

[59] Reddy DVS. 'The art of surgery in ancient India,' *Bull His Med,* vol. 6, 1938, pp. 81-87.

and cuts off his flesh making it equal to the weight of the dove, but on the scale his flesh remained lighter till he offered his whole body to the hawk. In this story from *Mahabharata* the services of a surgeon are not called for to surgically remove the flesh from the king's body. The moral of the story may be interpreted in many ways but this version probably has never been executed in any known sculpture from ancient times.

The other account is a Buddhist rendering telling a similar story without the involvement of other gods where the life of the dove was saved in exchange of king's own flesh. This story can be seen illustrated in two sculptures, one from about second century CE was discovered in Kosambi in Amarvati style and now exhibited in the National Museum of Madras (Chennai) India. The other is also a second century CE Gandhara relief which was discovered in a monastery in Swat (Pakistan) in 1910 (Fig. 8). This relief was first described in a paper published in 1913 as one of the finest examples of Gandhara sculptures and from the time. of its discovery it is in the British Museum.[60] The story on this Gandhara relief has been taken from a well known Jataka. The relief shows a dove which has taken refuge under the throne of King Sivi from the attack of the hawk. The king sitting under the canopy appears in distress being held by a female attendant, while another person or a surgeon holding a knife is kneeling as if cutting the flesh from the left leg of the king, behind the surgeon a standing figure is holding a weighing scale. There are two more celestial figures with halos standing and watching. At the canopy level may be seen an outline of a flying hawk although the figure is damaged and completely mutilated. As the story goes the hungry hawk demanded the prey he has been chasing and that he fully deserved his reward. In this Buddhist account it is implied that the Bodhisattva appearing as King Sivi

---

[60] Dames ML, Joyce TA. 'Note on a relief representing the story of Sivi,' *Man*, vol. 13, 1913, pp.17-10.

ordered his own flesh equal to the weight of the dove to be removed by a surgeon and given as food to the hawk thus saving the life of a helpless bird. The story is beautifully executed in this Gandhara sculpture.

From this sculpture we may also learn unrelated nevertheless interesting aspects of social life in Gandhara, for example it shows the kind of scales that was used for weighing purposes in Gandhara two thousands years ago. This type of weighing balance illustrated in this relief is known as steelyard or bismar, having a single pan, a graduated horizontal metal beam on which a sliding weight is moved. It was also a popular weighing device throughout the Roman Empire.[61] An example of such a balance from Roman period may be seen in British Museum. However in Gandhara weighing for the smaller amounts such as medicines or precious metals requiring precision weighing two pans hanging at the ends of a horizontal beam were generally used. The evidence lies in the weighing pans as small as 2.5 cm in diameter that have been excavated in Taxila and exhibited in the muscum.

Recently the archaeologists have discovered many rock carvings in the remote mountainous region of North Pakistan, among these one representing the Buddhist version of King Sivi story similar to the one described in the relief above was also discovered.[62] The Chinese traveller Fa Hien who had crossed these mountains from China into Swat must have visited the monastery where the above sculpture was housed or seen the rock carvings that have been discovered in 1994. Here is a quote from Fa Hien, which gives us an insight that he must have witnessed the relief or the rock carvings as related in the above story; his witness

---

[61] Derry TK, Williams TI. *A short history of technology*, Oxford: The Clarendon Press, 1960, pp. 222-23.

[62] Fussman G, Jettmar K, eds., *Antiquities of Northern Pakistan, reports and studies*, vol. 3, Mainz: Philips von Zabern, 1994, p.10.

also helps to accurately date these objects discovered in nineteenth century.[63]

> Seven day's journey thence the pilgrims arrived at the place where Sivika Raja delivered the dove.

The corroborated evidence contained in the above quote is not just an interesting episode it also brings out the fact that whenever the archaeological excavations get unexpected support from historical accounts both the historians and archaeologists get their rewards and such support allows them the opportunity of satisfaction that they have followed the right path.

The evidence about surgery that can be derived from the sculptures listed and discussed above is different what we have seen contained in the hymns of *Rig Veda*. The evidence cannot be considered a gold standard but at the same time it cannot be ignored altogether. Whatever has been mentioned above and some more to be seen below is indicative of prevailing concepts as regard to practice of surgery which, during later Buddhist period developed into more practical form.

There is one more piece of ancient object which is enthusiastically presented as a strong archaeological evidence of surgical practice in ancient India. This is a terracotta figure about which generally held view is that it belongs to 3rd or 4th century CE although no scientific investigation has been carried out to confirm its age. This curious specimen is the exhibit number 3175 in Allahabad museum, India (Fig.9). Although it is a crudely made clay structure and does not appear to carry any great artistic merit, since it represents a dissected human abdomen showing the viscera including

---

[63] Legge J. *A record of Buddhistic Kingdoms: being an account by the Chinese Monk Fa-Hien of his travels in India and Ceylon (AD 399-414) in search of Buddhist books of Discipline* (Reprint), New York: Paragon Book Reprint Corporation, 1965.

probably liver as well, it is judged to be revealing the story of a surgical procedure or illustrating some sort of medical theme. It is believed by some that this is not just a piece of oddity but an object indicative of social history of surgery or dissection. From the picture its craftsmanship looks poor and the whole structure is put together in an amateurish manner.

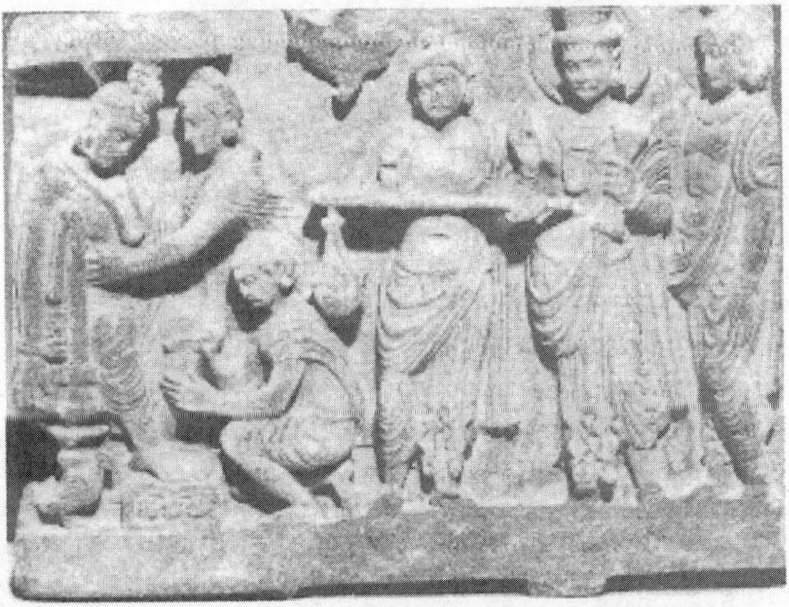

Fig. 8
The Gandhara sculpture where a surgeon is removing flesh from the thigh of the King Sivi, illustrating Sivi Jataka, British Museum.
(With kind permission of the Trustees of the British Museum, London).

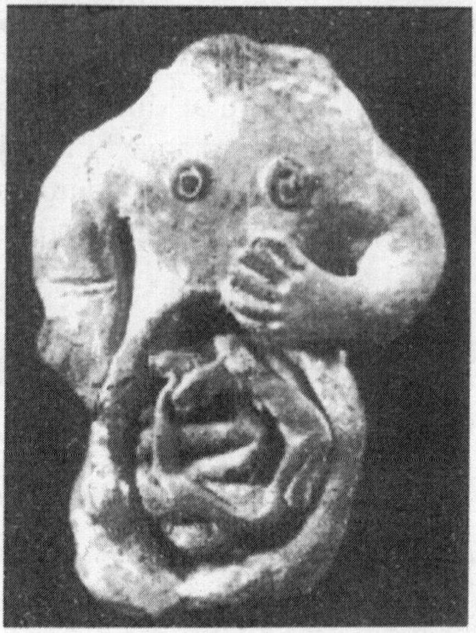

Fig. 9
Terracotta from 3rd-4th century CE showing dissected abdomen.
(With kind permission of Dr. S.K. Sharma, Director of the Allahabad Museum, Allahabad, India)

Unfortunately no serious investigation has been carried out to discover more about this odd and very strange looking figure from the past. The object has never been brought into any discussion or study in any wider forum of history of medicine. Probably further critical in depth study and investigation might result in its proper place in the history of surgery or dissection of human body. As regard to the origin of this only object of its kind there are two opinions; one explanation is that it was executed to celebrate the operation that Jivaka performed on a young boy who had developed abdominal complications and was cured by Jivaka's surgical intervention. The other speculation is that the object might have been designed as a teaching aid or a model showing the abdominal anatomy. Since it was discovered in Kosambi, a well known Buddhist territory in the past, the first opinion might be more likely and carry weight. This view may further be reinforced since the Jataka literature or the stories of Buddha's previous lives as

Bodhisattva were compiled about the time this terracotta has been alluded to.

Yet one more mythical story that has been put forward in evidence of surgery is contained in the *Jyotishka Jataka* where Buddha saved the life of an unborn child by delivering him from the womb of his dead mother. The story is from early life of Buddha when once he had given the good news to a mother predicting that she would give birth to a son, but a rival who wanted to prove Buddha wrong poisoned the woman who died. At her last rites for the cremation when the fire was lit to her pyre Buddha miraculously saved the unborn child, who was named Jyotishka meaning born of flames. Although there are different interpretations of this story, some have interpreted this miracle crediting Buddha to have delivered a live child by performing a caesarean operation on a dead woman. The sacred sculptures depicting this story are offered as further evidence of surgery. After all, many Buddhist scriptures such as *Mahavagga* the Buddha is also called Bhaisajya or Mahabhisak meaning the great doctor. Unlike the only two sculptures that illustrate the Sivi story, there are a number of Gandhara sculptures commemorating the miracle of birth of Jyotishka.[64] One relief shown here (Fig.10) is in the Lahore Museum, Pakistan. In this the central figure of a woman can be seen engulfed in flames and a child being removed from her side. Another, also a Gandhara sculpture, 40.5 x 37 cm is in Calcutta Museum also depicts the same story (accession number A23285). But the most beautiful sculpture of some artistic merit representing this story was carved in terracotta that was excavated in Afghanistan and was known to be in Kabul Museum, its fate after the recent turmoil remains unknown.

In the above account almost all sculptures that exist and reported in literature and according some support to surgery

[64] See note 33 above, pp. 525-27.

have been cited, while few have been illustrated in the above pages to give an opportunity to the readers to see the objects for themselves. The artistic elegance these objects bring out is no doubt is a great tribute to their creators, many were from Gandhara. How far they go to firmly establish the traditions of surgical practice in ancient times is most probably remains an open matter. The best course might be to leave to the individual readers to make their own minds, the facts and essential data has been put in front of them.

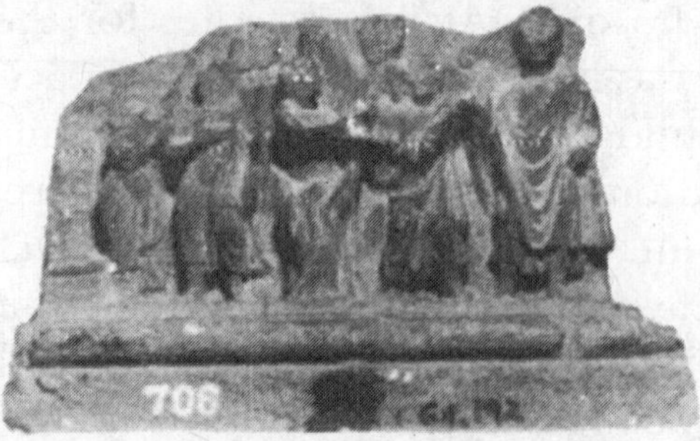

Fig. 10
A Gandhara relief telling the story of Jyotishka
(With kind permission of the Director of Lahore Museum, Lahore, Pakistan)

If we consider other purely epigraphic evidence from numerous edicts on stone, iron pillars and writings on plates of copper or silver that have been discovered during last two centuries we do not find any reference or suggestion in support of medical or surgical practice not only in Gandhara but any where else in the Indian subcontinent as well. One of the Ashoka's edicts quoted elsewhere; has recorded the cultivation of medicinal plants that bears a robust testimony of their use in the treatment of humans as well as animals but offers no support for surgical practice. In other words in support of surgical practice no convincing epigraphic evidence from ancient times has been discovered, published or ever been brought to light by the archaeologists in Gandhara or out side.

5.
The Birch Bark manuscripts from Gandhara

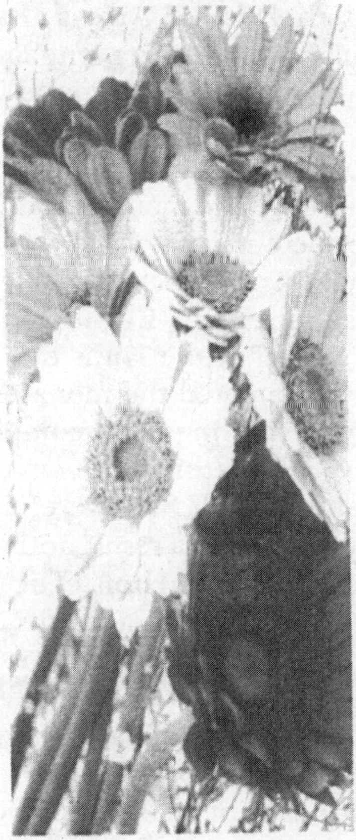

During the Buddhist supremacy in Gandhara if not political but religious capital always remained at Taxila. It was also a centre of academic activity for over a millennium where many historical figures the like of Atreya, Panini, Agnivesa, Nagarjuna and many more were engaged in scholastic pursue. With such pedagogic background of a capital city it is expected that textual remains will be discovered in abundance. Unfortunately this is not the case for which almost certainly there are two main reasons, both are equally factual. Firstly the medium of writing the texts available at the time was Birch Bark or probably palm leaves as well, both these materials are inherently fragile and easily perished. Secondly the invasion of White Huns that ended the glory of Gandhara for ever targeted the monasteries or Buddhist centres of learning, destroying them completely by burning thus eliminating all material in written form. The manuscripts written on Birch Bark were obviously far more easily destroyed by the fire, as a result nothing survived from the destructive zeal of White Huns. The evidence of this may be seen in the few charred fragments discovered in the monasteries. Few Birch Bark manuscripts that have been discovered were either discovered in the monasteries in remote inaccessible places in China or found in caves where they were possibly deposited by the monks out of reverence because sacred writings must not be destroyed. This tradition is practiced even today as regards to sacred books that are not used any more.

At this point it is cogent to have a detailed look and find out more about the nature of the birch bark; a common and popular material used for writing more than two millennium ago throughout Gandhara.

A Birch is a tree belonging to the genus *Betula* of which there are about 40 known species that grow at higher altitudes and in relatively cooler climate. In India and Pakistan it is variously known as *Bhurja, Sheetal, Kaidar, Padmal, Ghosh* or *Ghan*. The common feature of all birches is that they have wonderful bark with a variety of colours. In some species the bark can be peeled into large segments that can be shaped into flat leave like sheets. The bark of white birch or paper birch that is abundantly found in the valley of Kashmir was used as writing material in Gandhara and was known as *Bhurja patra* in Sanskrit. Its outer tough surface provides good protection while the inner smooth lightly coloured surface is used for writing with black ink. The ink is made from powdered charcoal and gum collected from trees, both were liquefied in water. The pens or styli were mostly shaped from dried bamboo, although a number of metal styli were also excavated from Taxila and are exhibited in the museum.

Alberuni in his *History of India* has given extremely useful and detailed account of how the birch bark was prepared in India for making books and similar other uses.[65]

> In Central and Northern India people use the bark of *Tuz* tree, one kind of which is used as a cover for bows. It is called Bhurja. They take piece one yard long and as broad as outstretched fingers of the hand or somewhat less, and prepare it in various ways. They oil and polish it so as to make it hard and smooth, and then they write on it. The proper order of single leaves is marked by numbers. The whole book is wrapped in a piece of cloth and fastened between two tablets of the same size. Such a book is called *puthi* (*pusta, pustaka*). Their letters or whatever they have to write, they write on the bark of the *Tuz* tree.

This is an admirable piece of history written expressively by an eye witness. In Taxila only few fragments of birch bark manuscripts were discovered from the site at the Dharmarajika which are exhibited in the museum, three

[65] See note 17 above, p. 171.

are illustrated here (Fig.11. Their writing is in Brahmi script and these fragments were dated to fifth century CE. The few words when deciphered by the epigraphists indicate that they must have come from a Buddhist scripture and show no indication of medical origin. From another monastery at Jaulian in Taxila about 53 fragments were discovered in an earthenware jar, these were also badly damaged by the fire, what little writing remained showed that the script and subject matter was of similar in nature as those 3 fragments discussed above.[66] The present where about of these 53 segments is not known?

However during late nineteenth and twentieth centuries a number of birch bark manuscripts, some complete others incomplete were discovered in other places with in Gandhara and also from the ruined monasteries along the Silk Road. Few of these are medical while majority are Buddhist scriptures. The early discoveries mostly around Khotan or present day Xinjiang province of China by the French, German, Russian, Swedish, Japanese and British archaeological adventurers were all properly documented and now held at the well known museums or academic institutions. The best known collector of these and other antiquities was Aurel Stein (1862-1943) who made many hazardous journeys into inaccessible deserts and brought with him camel loads of valuable Buddhist antiques and manuscripts which were deposited in British Museum.[67]

In the last decade of the twentieth century few other birch bark scrolls from the second century CE preserved in clay jars were acquired from private collectors by the British Library and University of Washington in Seattle, these have now been deciphered under eminent scholars.[68] Their origin

---

[66] See note 33 above, pp. 287-88 and 387.

[67] Walker A. *Aurel Stein: Pioneer of the Silk Road*, London: John Murray, 1995.

[68] Solomon R. 'The Senior Manuscripts: Another collection of Gandhara Buddhist Scrolls', *Journal of the American Oriental Society,* 2003; 123.1: pp. 73-92.

and time of discovery and by who is still a mystery and wrapped up in suspicions. These manuscripts are collectively known as Gandhari Scrolls and have been compared to the Dead Sea Scrolls both in the mystery surrounding their discovery and historical importance being the earliest documents ever come to light from the Buddhist period. Since these are now in academic control not many eye brows are raised. They were written in a language the modern experts have labelled Gandhari which previously was known as Prakrit, a form of regional Sanskrit which was simpler and less complicated grammatically than classical Sanskrit. It was the language widely used throughout Gandhara for centuries and written in Kharoshthi script. The Kharoshthi script heavily borrowed from the Aramaic alphabet that was perhaps a legacy from the Achaemenian conquest of Gandhara. These recently re-discovered, investigated and translated scrolls are all about Buddhist scriptures and none relates to medical or surgical subjects. In contrast some of the earlier finds were purely on secular subjects and some were probably written as medical texts for the purpose of teaching or reference books for the Monks residing in monasteries in isolated places. Many of the manuscripts we have today were discovered from the sites along the Silk Road, while most were written in a non classical Sanskrit language typical of Gandhara style.

The most important of these is known as the *Bower Manuscript* and a brief discussion on this exceptional medical manuscript along with the other major three medical treatises will follow. Such an approach must be useful because the *Bower Manuscript* is the only medical manuscript ever discovered completely and its originality lends tremendous support to the others. The *Bower Manuscript* will be examined before discussing the well known medical texts of *Caraka Samhita* and *Susruta Samhita*. Such an approach will make better sense to bring about the proposition that the earliest medical texts were the result of the contributions of the writers from Gandhara and later by those who travelled from Gandhara to the monasteries on the road to China.

This arrangement may not comply with the chronological norm but it is desirable because the *Bower Manuscript* is the only authentic complete manuscript written on birch bark comes to us as a reliable source that also underpins the other texts which are anterior to it. This role of authentication the *Bower Manuscript* plays places it in an important and unique position.

Apart from the medical birch bark manuscripts the earliest and oldest mathematical manuscript written on the birch bark was also discovered in Gandhara. It is known as *Bakhshali Manuscript* because it was discovered in the village called Bakhshali near to Peshawar in 1881. It is also written in non classical Sanskrit in a script that was used by the Buddhist of Gandhara. The authorship cannot be ascertained while it has been variously dated from 4th century CE to about 7th CE. The manuscript employs the decimal place value and it is in fact a commentary on mathematical works of earlier period. Consisting of seventy leaves the *Bakhshali Manuscript* is also housed at the Bodleian Library of the Oxford University. The date of this mathematical manuscript may not be known accurately but its discovery in Gandhara further strengths the notion that Gandhara remained cradle for all sciences and a basic discipline such as mathematics was an essential part of this learning.

Fig. 11

Fragments of charred Birch Bark manuscript in Taxila museum

6.
The Bower Manuscript

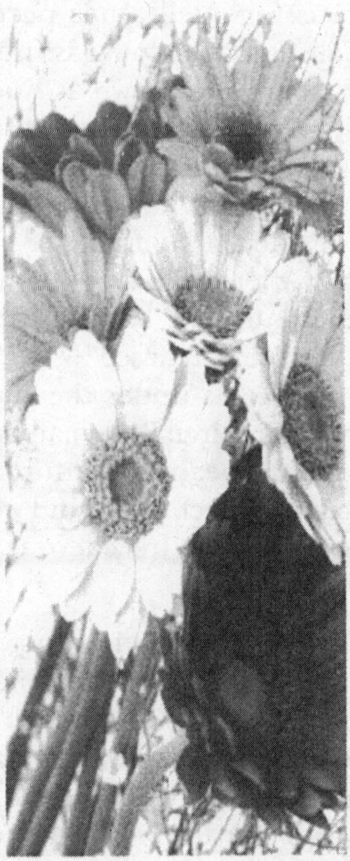

The first complete and the only original Buddhist medical manuscript ever discovered is known as the *Bower Manuscript,* after the person who first purchased it. In about 1888 a British army lieutenant Hamilton Bower was perusing in remote Xinjiang province of China an Afghan, who had murdered an English businessman. His other purpose was to collect and establish contacts for intelligence purposes to stall off the Russian Imperialist advance towards India. While he was in a place called Kucher now known as Kuqa an oasis town of ancient Buddhist monasteries on the Silk Road he purchased 51 leaves of a Birch Bark manuscript. In 1890 this manuscript ultimately reached in the hands of the great palaeographer A.F. Rudolph Hoernle (1841-1918) who was professor at Calcutta. After the translation and editing work was completed the manuscript was returned to the owner and later it was acquired or purchased by the Bodleian Library at Oxford, where it remains under the catalogue number 1090. The discovery of this Birch Bark manuscript also started a race among many Europeans adventurers as mentioned above, who competed with each other and with great secrecy; passion and gusto travelled the treacherous deserts of China in search of such treasurers.

Hoernle published its translation first in a number of instalments between 1893-1912 and finally a complete translation was published in a folio format.[69] It was estimated by Hoernle that the manuscript was written around the third quarter of fourth century CE, but now it is agreed that the correct date must be first half of sixth century CE. Its language is Sanskrit written in Nagari script but the language

[69] See note 49 above.

is not classical Sanskrit it is mixed with local dialects. The translator in the introduction has also argued that it is essentially a product of North India or Gandhara and also the birch bark it is written on originated from Kashmir.[70] The physical nature of the leaves as described by Hoernle indicates that it might have been prepared in difficult circumstances, for example the leaves are not of highest quality whereas the scarcity was to the extent that even a badly damaged and tattered leaf was also employed. The shape of leaves is oblong approximately 65 cm in length and 7 cm wide, having a hole on one side for the string to keep all together. Most Birch Bark manuscripts are quadrangular in shape and have central whole for the string. May be some Buddhist monks from Gandhara prepared it during the period when the monasteries were stuck with poverty. It was probably written as a medical guide at Kuqa where it was discovered in unknown circumstances in the late nineteenth century. Such a speculation may hold some plausibility if we consider that the turmoil in Gandhara and persecution of the Buddhism during and after the invasion of the White Huns lasted for a long period of time resulting in completely annihilation of Buddhism from Gandhara. Owing to extremely violent state of affairs the Buddhist monks were forced to migrate; finding refuge in remote places in conditions of great hardship and desolation. The manuscript does show the name of a monk called Yasometra and the monastery where it was found was dedicated to him. What limited information available about the *Bower Manuscript* it is impossible to pinpoint the real authors, correct place of the origin and absolutely accurate date of this hugely informative and the only medical manuscript of its kind ever came to light.

From the comprehensive critical study of the *Bower Manuscript* as carried out by its translator and editor we can derive great deal of interesting information relevant to the practice of medicine in Gandhara though nothing on surgery.

---

[70] See note 49 above, p. xlviii.

This is probably because it was intended to be a text primarily on therapeutics and internal medicine for the use in a remote monastery. Another reason for surgery not mentioned may be that the art of surgery had died by the time the text of the *Bower Manuscript* was compiled. The manuscript seems to have been written not by a single author but at least three or even four different persons. It is written with a pen shaped from reed and not a brush, a sure evidence of its non Chinese origin. There are references to a number of medical authorities who are mentioned with devout respect and reverences. Among these Atreya is mentioned as the great teacher in Taxila and at least 6 prescriptions are cited after him. About 12 formulae are from Bhela, who is also revered. Then Caraka himself is repeatedly mentioned and nearly 29 formulae or preparations are recorded that have been borrowed from him, these are also seen in the *Caraka Samhita.* Similarly great respect is conferred to Susruta from whom about 6 prescriptions are borrowed. But unfortunately no surgical aspect as contained in the present *Susruta Samhita* is recorded in the *Bower Manuscript.* The last authority from old times adoringly referred to in the *Bower Manuscript* is Vagbhata. The references to these authorities are not to their texts but by their names whenever any prescription is borrowed. It looks that during the time of the writers of the *Bower manuscript* these works may not be available although the oral traditions were alive. The real value and importance of the *Bower Manuscript* lies in the fact that this is the only manuscript came to us in its original and complete form. All other medical texts were manifestly products of gross changes and additions by those who re-wrote them at much later date. The allusions in the *Bower Manuscript* of some of the names unfortunately give us no clue if any such texts existed during the time or before the *Bower Manuscript* was compiled.

The *Bower Manuscript* also records a number of chants and invocations or mantras that are to be invoked for various medical or other situations. But when we consider purely medical aspects we find interesting details throwing light on the Buddhist medicine of the time. The first full chapter is on the medical uses and benefits of garlic depicted as *lasuna (Lhassan* in current usage). This chapter has found special popularity among those who have written critical accounts about the *Bower Manuscript.* There are also a number of recipes for food preparations with garlic as the major constituent. It is important to note that the garlic is recommended to be cooked with various meats. The *Bower Manuscript* gives great importance to garlic as an herb which is full of health restoring properties. Despite the age old Brahmanic prohibition against garlic the *Bower Manuscript* ingeniously advocates that even Brahmans can derive benefits from it by first feeding the garlic to the cows and then consuming their milk or milk products.

The pharmacy of the agents that have been recorded by the writers of the *Bower Manuscript* provides the most interesting correlation with some of the artefacts excavated in Gandhara and these might have been used in the preparations of many pharmaceutical preparations. It is a perfectly logical assumption that in order to prepare the compound medicines and other preparations in this manuscript a variety of equipment must be available not only to prepare but to store them in some kind of containers or medicine jars for transportation and hand over to the patients in viable condition.

In the following list a selection of the groups of medical preparations that have been recorded in the *Bower Manuscript* are recorded, although the list given below is by no means complete. Similar names may also be seen in the other three Samhitas as well. This catalogue of therapeutic agents that is common among almost all the major medical texts offers us some understanding regarding the vast numbers of therapeutic agents available to the physicians of the time. The number of prepared items included in Ayurvedic practice was huge which required extensive range of pharmaceutical equipment like weighing balances, measuring jars and many other devices, their existence can be corroborated from the archaeological discoveries in Gandhara.

Pills	Potions
Decoctions	Elixirs
Inhalants	Smoking
Eye drops	Collyrium
Poultices	Lotions
Unguents	Medicated oils
Tampons	Powders
Medicated Bandages	Douches
Cotton swabs	Purgatives
Suppositories	Fomentation
Enemas	Emetics
Gargles	Anti aging agents
Aphrodisiacs	

It is obvious that these agents must be prepared, stored, dispensed and occasionally administered with the help of some kind of equipment or instruments. As mentioned above a number of such instruments have also been excavated at various sites in Gandhara and more so in Taxila. Some of these may be seen catalogued by Sir John Marshall while others excavated afterwards are on display in various showcases. But unfortunately the related items are not exhibited in an orderly manner so that seemingly medically related items may be placed together along with relevant information or appropriate labelling. Such organised display probably requires great deal of research of each individual exhibit and no doubt entails academic efforts as well as resources. However the presence of many of these pharmaceutical related objects in Taxila museum obviously puts across glaringly the long association of Taxila with health care. The teaching about medicinal plants was an important aspect of the medical education.

The *Bower Manuscript* is unique in many respects, e.g. its use of various measures and weights to carefully determine accurate quantities of the medicinal constituents in the preparation of various prescriptions or formulae for pills, powders or poultices and numerous other preparations offers extremely useful data. The weighing of smaller quantity also necessitated utilization of small enough pans for the weighing scales or weighing balances, which have been excavated and such small pans or scales are among the exhibits. This kind of collaboration between the textual accounts recorded in the *Bower Manuscript* and relevant exhibits in the museum not only offers interesting reading but can also bestow mutual validation. This aspect will be further elaborated in the last chapter.

At this stage it will be apt to examine just one method of administration of various medications that have been listed above and talk about what kind of equipment the pharmacists of Taxila might have used to dispense these prepared substances to their patients. Although the *Bower Manuscript* is not the only one in listing medicated inhalants as cure for different conditions others have also described this method. A tubing crafted from a bamboo or other hollow stem of a suitable plant has been advocated to be used for inhalation of smoke produced by the burning of various medicated substances. There is a mention of an earthen ware pot in *Caraka Samhita;* it seems to be a device consisting of two pieces, which was recommended for the use of medicated inhalants after evaporating by putting the pots on fire.[71] Administering some medicines by Inhaling has been described in *Caraka Samhita, Susruta Samhita* and also in Vagbhata's *Astangasangraha* as well. The *Bower Manuscript* in the treatment of coryza (common cold) has advised the following inhalational treatment; where according to the translator of the grains is not legible in the original leave of the *Bower Manuscript.*[72]

[71] Caraka Samhita VI, xxi.

[72] See note 49 above, p.130.

> The patient may also inhale the fumes produced from powdered grains ... well mixed with clarified butter made to burn in a crucible covered with a lid.

Among the multitudes of pottery items that have been excavated in Taxila, it is not difficult in majority of cases to imagine the purpose and practical uses of these items in day today life. However there is one very strange piece that is curious and unusual. It is a jug shaped red clay pottery with narrow rimmed mouth, robust handle, and flat bottom having four spouts clustered together on one side. It is nearly six inches or about 15 cm in height and was excavated from the stratum II at Bhir Mound site in Taxila. Sir John Marshall in his catalogue has not given any archaeological assessment or comments as to its use or the purpose or comments for quaintness of four spouts.[73] This piece of pottery is uniquely different than many other exhibited in the museum. Its four spouts and narrow neck strongly suggest it might have been the kind of inhaler described in the texts mentioned above. When placed side by side with a nineteenth century inhaler it is plain simple to imagine that the inhalants mentioned by the authors of the *Bower Manuscript* and other texts might have been dispensed, with such an earthenware pot. The design of this pottery fits well into the scheme because at least one use for this we can think off is as an inhaler and no other possible uses can be envisaged. Its size is just right, positioning of the four spouts near to each other and the height at which the spouts are sited also looks right so that the medicated vapours will be efficiently available for inhalation purpose, especially if the head of the patient and the inhaler are both covered with some sort of cloth or suitable fabric. Similar method was frequently recommended by the medical profession about the middle of nineteenth century when a variety of special stoneware were introduced for dispensing inhalants mixed with very hot water and inhaling the vapours rising through its spout. One such device known

[73] See note 33 above, vol. ii, p. 415.

as Dr. Nelson's inhaler manufactured for this purpose may still be seen (Fig. 12). These inhalers are often seen in medical antique shops and are popular collecting items. Moreover even today the teachers who train the young singers recommend to their pupils inhalation of medicated substances from similar inhaler as seen on the left in the picture that can be purchased as an accessory from some of the music shops or pharmacies. When placed side by side there is remarkable similarity both in the design and the function of these inhalers, one is couple of thousand years older than the other.

The sections IV and V of the *Bower Manuscript* do not deal with medicine, these two chapters talk about totally different kind of subject altogether. It is obvious that these two chapters were definitely not written by the same author or authors who wrote the medical chapters of the *Bower Manuscript*. The chapters or sections IV and V touch on magic and deal with fortune telling. It seems obvious there is exploitation of psychic of the people who must had firm belief in supernatural powers.

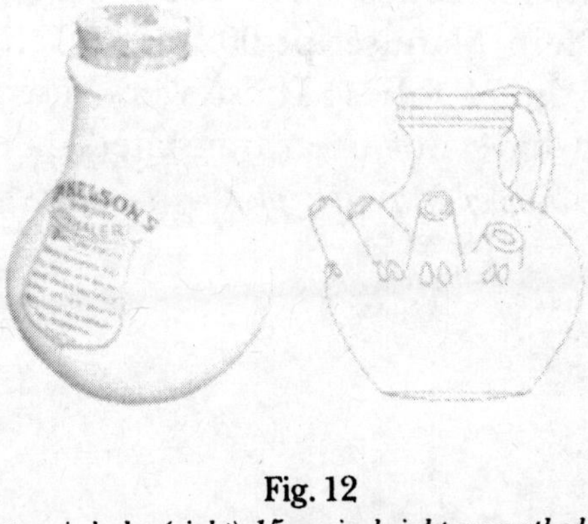

Fig. 12

A four spouted pottery inhaler (right) 15 cm in height unearthed in Taxila, compared with a mid 19th century inhaler known as Dr. Nelson's Inhaler, about 20 cm in height.

A number of other objects displayed in the Taxila museum that appear as pharmaceutical objects and might had been used for numerous preparations that have been mentioned in the *Bower Manuscript,* would be taken into consideration at a later stage when rest of the surgical instruments and medical equipment will be discussed below.

Although the *Bower Manuscript* is the most important and significant manuscript ever discovered most probably originated from Gandhara, there are few others so called minor medical manuscripts that were discovered when an exhaustive search was undertaken in Eastern Turkistan after the discovery of the *Bower Manuscript.* Most are not considered particularly of high value; some are not even complete and were found only in fragments and have not been studied or even translated with the same zeal as the *Bower Manuscript.* Moreover their contents are also not strictly dealing with medicine. These are about magical, spells, charms or religious incantations. In comparison to the *Bower Manuscript* the scientific value of these so called minor medical manuscripts is lot poorer.

A number of other Birch Bark manuscripts are also discussed by Hoernle, among them only few have been labelled as medical manuscripts but all of these are fragments or consist of only few folios.[74] The two medical manuscripts are known as Stein Manuscript 002 in 65 folios and Stein Manuscript 003 in 71 folios. These were discovered by Sir Aural Stein and have not been translated or edited in the same way as the *Bower Manuscript.*

---

[74] Hoernle AFR. ed., *Manuscript remains of Buddhist literature found in Eastern Turkistan,* Amsterdam: Philo Press, 1970.

7.
Gandhara and the medical compendiums

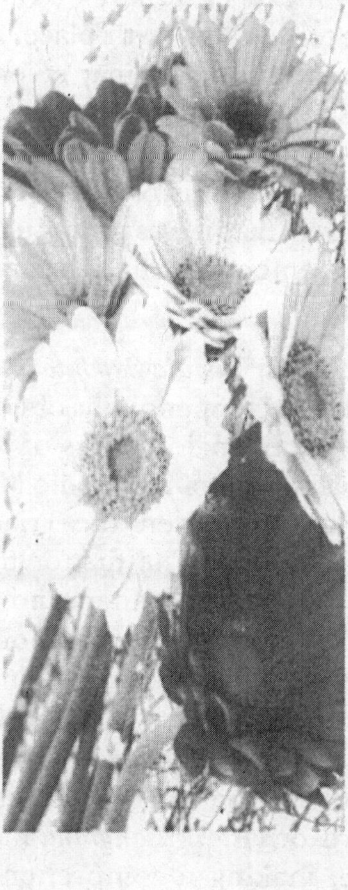

In Gandhara Taxila remained a centre for learning and education most likely from the Vedic times till the decline of Buddhist civilisation. If it is accepted that the earliest renderings of the medical compendiums of Caraka and Susruta belong to an age bordering the Vedic period then inevitably these two texts must have originated in Gandhara and Taxila ought to be their birth place. As a consequence of such an argument a scenario may be envisaged based on the historical upshot that requires us to consider that the roots of the three Samhitas discussed below must lay in Gandhara. As regard the origin of *Bower Manuscript* no further argument is required that it was a product of Gandhara, its contents and style embodies enough facts to demonstrate its Gandhara origin.

The *Caraka Samhita, Susruta Samhita* and *Astangasangraha* or in simple words the compendiums of Caraka, Susruta and Vagbhata are the three major works of medicine that are considered the back bone of Ayurvedic Medicine. They are referred by the Sanskrit writers the Triad (*trayi*) or three great writings in medicine. The first or the *Caraka Samhita* notably encompasses what we understand internal medicine with only minimal or mere passing mention of surgery. While the second or *Susruta Samhita* is unique in the exposition of surgical treatments and portrayal of the tools used in the practice of surgery. The medicine contained in the *Susruta Samhita* is more or less on the same lines as in the *Caraka Samhita*. The third or *Astangasangraha* has combined both the fields in one, making a comprehensive text book of general medicine and surgery. How the Gandharian School or the Buddhist medical intelligent influenced or contributed directly or indirectly in these three most fundamental works of Ayurveda is to be discussed in this chapter.

If a connection is to be sought linking these texts with Gandhara it must centre and take into consideration the time and period of each of these. But any discussion on the dates or time particularly the first two texts is full of difficulties and problems because there are multitudes of claims recorded in the whole host of publications by authors with over zealous disputations regarding the period of the first two Samhitas. As an example the most comprehensive publication on the subject of the history of Indian medicine by Meulenbeld there are 270 references on the period of *Caraka Samhita* alone, which give as many views about the time of the text and its author. Further in the same publication over fifty references allocate to Caraka a period from 100 CE to well over 1000 BCE.[75] Thousands of years BCE is not an uncommon statement seen in quite few of these publications. This also means sieving through such divergent views makes it difficult to reach at any rational conclusion. This situation presents further difficulties if historians should waste their efforts and time of their audience by merely filling pages with unbelievable assertions that are simply far beyond the conventional norms.

Traditionally both in Greek and Indian mythology only gods had the knowledge of medicine who for the love of humanity handed this sacred knowledge over to selected godly human beings. The mythology ends as soon as this heavenly insight into cure of diseases was handed over to those earthly beings who were the first interface between gods and humans. The wisdom was memorised and further disseminated mostly from father to the sons or the teacher to the trusted loyal pupils. Eventually it was recorded in sacred texts written on palm leaves, birch bark and similar

[75] See note 14 above, vol. IB, p.184 and vol. IA, p.115.

other perishable materials. The unfolding of the events in this way offers a fair compromise between those who must continue believing in mythology and others with secular disposition. But as we arrive at this amicable arrangement the problems begins for the historiographers of the Indian medical history. They find it difficult to track down any trace of chronology or source material acceptable to their yard sticks. The *Bower Manuscript* as described above is the only reliable and original source that throws some muted light. As regard Caraka we find references that he must be a physician, while Chinese sources tell that a physician of the same name happened to be serving in the court of Kanishka.[76] Here we may find some plausible explication for the historiographers to satisfy their methodologies though the inconsistencies in historical narratives are not fully satisfactory.

In summary if we apply the above notions to the *Caraka Samhita,* the myths tell us that gods imparted the knowledge of medicine to Atreya, who was teacher in Taxila, he passed on the knowledge to his six pupils, among them Agnivesa was one who most probably memorised the teachings of the great teacher and then passed on to the next generation. This sequence of events may be gleamed as recorded by convention in most writings. At some point in time enters the factual historical figure who was Kanishka's physician by the name of Caraka, whose feats as skilled obstetrician saving Kanishka's wife during difficult childbirth have been recorded in a nineteenth century German source though discounted by others.[77] Caraka some times during the reign of Kanishka recounted the text that Agnivesa had preserved in whatever form or at an unknown period, while we are in total darkness about the long period between Agnivesa and Caraka. Unfortunately the Caraka's revision of Agnivesa's

[76] Wujastyk D. *The roots of Ayurveda,* New Delhi: Penguin Books, 2001, p. 40.

[77] See note 43 above, pp.1-12.

original work remains obscure and elusive, only its name crops up but no definite citing has been found in any text. Still from these shadows emerges one more and final personality with the name of Dridabala, about him the first author who gives us some information in English was probably Hoernle.[78] Dridabala on his own count more or less completely revised the original work of Caraka. We are also told that he belonged to a family of famous physicians but as regard the precise age he flourished there is no firm agreement. A possible period when he might have lived has been quoted by Chattopadhyaya is 3rd or 4th century CE.[79] While others have stated 4th to 5th CE, but Hoernle after analyzing the references from a number of medical writings and making a comprehensive chronological study of all the writers connected with *Caraka Samhita* and *Susruta Samhita,* has placed Dridabala during 7th to 8th century CE. A span of 4th to 8th CE is fairly long period that can create uncertainties. As for as Caraka's association with Taxila is concerned not many serious alternative opinions have ever been proposed. On the other hand Dridabala has been described to belong to a locality called Panchanada (also written as Pancanada) in Kashmir at the meeting place of the River Jhelum and Indus by Hoernle, as in the following statement that he interpreted from Dridabala's own statement.[80]

> It is this Kashmirian Panchanada, which probably was the home of Dridabala.

After making this statement with piquant use of 'probably' Hoernle tried desperately to locate Panchanada by making an additional observation in the foot note. Because he himself never lived in the North he employed the help of Aural Stein to find the where about of Panchanada. But

---

[78] Hoernle AFR. *Studies in the medicine of ancient India, Part I. Osteology or the bones of the human body,* Oxford: The Clarendon Press, 1907, pp. 7-17.

[79] See note 22 above, p. 32.

[80] See note 78 above, pp. 7-17.

it seems from what is recorded in the footnote they were both talking about a place named Panjpur in the district of Attock and not Panchanada. However there is a small township known as Pachnand situated approximately at 32.5N and 72.5E, about 150 miles south of Taxila. This place can equally be speculated to be a probable place of Dridabala's abode as mentioned and quoted by Hoernle. This place no doubt was within the boundaries of Gandhara and may be under the influence of Kashmir when Dridabala prospered and claimed to be Kashmirian. This information can easily connect the original *Caraka Samhita* and its later reviser Dridabala to Gandhara. In order to clarify and steer clear from confusion we need to keep the following points in mind.

1. Panchanada meaning five rivers was an ancient Sanskrit name of the province of the Panjab (spellings recommended by the University of the Panjab). The *Mahabharata* and *Ramayana* both have used this name. The Panjab (five waters) was the literal Persian translation from Sanskrit name of Panchanada, which was introduced much later by the Muslims but became popular and prevalent.

2. Panchanada sometimes identifies confluence of two or more rivers and traditionally such a place acquires a sacred entity known as Tirath. In Indian music Panchanada is also used to portray a form of music or a specific musical instrument.

3. It is a myth and denial of geography what has been recorded by Hoernle and repeated by others that the River Indus and the River Jhelum meet at a place called Panchanada in Kashmir.[81] The fact is they run at a distance of more than 200 miles from each other and only meet once other three rivers are also joined further in south after running a course of hundreds

[81] See note 22 above, p. 31.

of miles at a place called today as Pachnad (five rivers), this place was identified by Alberuni as Panchanada and Alberuni has also used this name to represent one of the countries in the West, obviously the province of Panjab.[82] If Dridabala came from this place even then his connection with Gandhara remains undisputed because this was also part of Gandhara.

4. Both in Persian and Sanskrit languages the word 'panj' is analogous, meaning five and in both languages the terminology has been employed in a variety of expressions or creating pun both in prose and poetry.

On the other hand Dridabala's association with Kashmir may also be factual, if we consider the historical realities during the period Dridabala might have existed, when the whole of Gandhara was in turmoil following the White Hun invasion. It is quite logical that at this time Kashmir was relatively safe place of refuge where people from Gandhara might have moved for safety sake. It is likely that Dridabala's link with Gandhara as contended above may appear speculative but it is as plausible as many other inconsistencies that have been recorded by many and accepted in the historical accounts of the period.

We can never find out all the sources oral or written that Dridabala had to his disposal at the time he started to revise and adding to the original text of *Caraka Samhita.* Moreover we are also not sure about the validity of the final revision by Dridabala, because no original manuscript has ever been discovered. In this respect it is noteworthy what Manfred Ullman has recorded that during the reign of Khosrow I (reigned 531-579 CE) his doctor Burzoe had travelled to India and brought back *Pancatantra* and some medical books as well. *Pancatantra* literally means five chapters; is the famous book of fables that was translated

---

[82] See note 17 above, p. 260 and p. 302.

into Pehlvi (Old Persian) and then into Syriac and in 8th CE into Arabic. From this Arabic translation it was preserved in Latin and other European languages while the original Sanskrit version has been lost. Although Ullman does not elaborate what medical books Burzoe brought back but it is unthinkable if *Caraka Samhita* was not among them. This also makes it highly probable that Burzoe must have brought with him the edition of *Caraka Samhita* that was redacted by Dridabala. Additionally the following quote from Ullman throws more light and offers further details.[83]

> The *Caraka Samhita,* a medical compendium that contains the teachings of Agnivesa, was to the account of Ibn-an- Nadim, first translated from Indian into Persian and then translated further into Arabic by a certain Abd Allah ibn Ali...... . Ali Ibn Sahl at Tabari, in the appendix to his *Kitab Firdaws al Hikma* (850 CE) has given an expose of the system of Indian medicine. Ali has in this relied on the Persian or Arabic translation of the books of Caraka, Susruta, Vagbhata and Madhavakara.

Since no original Sanskrit manuscripts have ever been discovered it is probable that the present *Caraka Samhita* and *Susruta Samhita* were only saved in the same way as many other Greek and Indian works because they were translated into Persian or Arabic.

The story of *Caraka Samhita* as related above commencing with mythology and through intermediaries reached to its last contributor Dridabala who in turn gave us the present or the final edition of *Caraka Samhita.* This sequence of events establishes that the text is wholly a product of Gandhara School. The fact that its origin was rooted in Taxila has also been alluded to by the modern historian of standing.[84]

---

[83] Ullman M. *Islamic medicine.* Edinburgh: Edinburgh University Press, 1978, pp. 19-20. Also see Brown EG. *Arabian Medicine,* Cambridge: The University Press, 1921, p. 21.

[84] Porter R. *The greatest benefit to mankind,* London: Harper Collins, 1977. p. 138.

Now we look into the journey in time of *Susruta Samhita,* which is a compendium dealing with surgery and no doubt stands in unique position, the only other available and comparable text might be the *De Medicina* of the mid first century CE compiled by the Roman surgeon Celsus. As in case of *Caraka Samhita* the Indian authors have allocated dates to *Susruta Samhita* from 3000 BCE to the last few centuries BCE, this absurd span of dating has been mentioned by many authors and few references that have claimed this have been cited at appropriate places.

The *Susruta Samhita* is not mentioned by any medical or non medical source from antiquity; even the two Samhitas of Caraka and Susruta do not mention each other. The first authentic medical text that refers it is the *Bower Manuscript,* which in fact has copied few prescriptions from it as well, with due acknowledgement. It seems during its development *Susruta Samhita* also passed similar stages as we have noticed with *Caraka Samhita.* For example during the early period of development of *Susruta Samhita* the involvement of gods and myths surrounding it is even greater. The mythological starting point of this text begins when a number of eminent gods or saints gathered at a sacred unknown place in the high mountains. Among them was Dhanvantari who had received the wisdom from higher divine sources and descends to earth as Divadosa to teach the art of surgery to his pupil Susruta. Similarity with Atreya and his pupil Agnivesa are obvious. At the end of each chapter as in *Caraka Samhita* the *Susruta Samhita* also acknowledges the teacher with salutations paying apt respects to the honourable Dhanvantari or Divadosa. The book also acknowledges additional great teacher *Kasiraja* or the king of Kashi (or Benares). This presents a historical quandary whether he was a real king or his pupil bestowing an honour out of immense respect to the teacher. The narrative remains in the realm of myths as there seems to be no historical veracity for a king of this name ever ruled Kashi although this perception has conferred to *Susruta Samhita* the ethnicity of Kashi. After meticulous search Hoernle records the following statement regarding the date of Susruta; however others entirely disagree with him.[85]

> Regarding the date of Susruta we have the following indication. He must have been acquainted with the doctrine of Atreya. With reference for example to the bones of the human body, he introduces his own exposition with a remark pointing out the difference between Atreya's system and his own in respect of the total number of the bones. This proves that Susruta cannot have been anterior to Atreya...... . The probability therefore, appears to be that Susruta was a rather younger contemporary of Atreya, or let us say a contemporary of Atreya's pupil Agnivesa.

This argument assigns approximate period of Susruta in the sixth century BCE but we are still in dark and are deemed to remain so as to his place of residence. On the other hand Keswani has placed the historical Susruta in the second century BCE, but has not gone into the discussion regarding the place where Susruta might have come from.[86] It has also been pointed out that any wise man who knew many cures was called Susruta and there were a number of people known as Susruta at different periods of history. It is also possible people adopted the name to seek popularity.

Turning to other opinions we also come across those who believe there was no single author of *Susruta Samhita,* the justification given for this is because there are enormous amount of facts accumulated in the single text, which must be the result of efforts of multiple writers. This also renders the search for a single writer futile and to seek out for a historical Susruta becomes nothing but frustratingly vain effort. As for as Kasiraja is concerned one authority of repute

[85] See note 78 above, p. 8

[86] Keswani NH, ed., *The science of medicine and physiological conceptions in ancient and medieval India.,* New Delhi: All India Institute of Medical Sciences, 1974, p.13.

Fazilliot, in his much referred book chooses not to mention the story of *Kasiraja* altogether. After making a detailed argument and analysis of literature the author makes the statement that seems to be accepted and agreed by most other writers.[87]

> The personage of Susruta not being historical, the *Susruta Samhita* shows itself to be not as the personal work of a certain Susruta, but as the anonymously edited manual of certain school which had selected a Susruta for patron. We know by the very tradition of this school, that this manual has reached us after having touched at least once. The commentator Dalhana (xi-xii century AD) affirms in effect that Nagarjuna has been the reconstructor of the Susruta Samhita.

A surprising aspect is that during a long period extending many centuries before it was reconstructed by Nagarjuna, this surgical treatise was supposedly prevalent but no other source secular or religious had ever made any reference to it or to its author. Another vital problem that becomes noticeable on critical analysis is that evidence of practice of surgery as advance and organized as recorded in *Susruta Samhita* is also not supported by any other literary testimony. On the other hand the religious scruples in relation to the rituals in respect of untouchables had actually resulted in the discouragement of surgery. In these circumstances a firm evidence to assign a period for the origin of *Susruta Samhita* seems to be an impossible task.

The testimony of surgical practice during the Buddhist monastic period in Taxila is undoubtedly evident and may be verified form the surgical implements that were excavated from the sites of well known monasteries. Moreover these artefacts start appearing from the layers starting from the time of Ashoka and reach the peak during first two centuries of the first millennium. We also notice that there have been no discoveries of such items before and after this window of

---

[87] See note 45 above, p.14.

few centuries. This was also the period when the advancement of Buddhist sciences was at the peak. The historical evidence in support of this premise may be derived from number of names of the scientists and their literary contributions during the same period. As an example the final commentator or editor of *Susruta Samhita,* Misra Dalhana has pointed to the name of Nagarjuna being the author of the doctrine contained in what we know as *Susruta Samhita.* About this Nagarjuna another historian Kutumbiah gives us the following information.[88]

> There exists an Indian tradition which assigns the revised and supplemented edition of Susruta's original work to Nagarjuna. If he should be the well-known Buddhist patriarch of that name, who is said to have been the contemporary of King Kanishka, his date would practically coincide with that of Caraka. Accordingly the original compendia of Agnivesa and Susruta should have been revised and re-edited at much the same time.

Nagarjuna has been briefly mentioned above in respect of Mahayana Buddhism (the Greater Vehicle), to which he was the major contributor during the time of Kanishka. The other major contribution of this all round talented courtier in Kanishka's court was the compilation of the surgical manual that later became known as *Susruta Samhita,* while other philosophical contributions of Nagarjuna are out side the scope of present discussion and cannot be listed or fully discussed here. But his intellect was quite capable to have completely written the *Susruta Samhita* even if such a text did not exist before him. This compilation was a crucial development after which the text seems to emerge into a reality containing rational concepts and eventually found its place as a legitimate text of medicine and surgery. Although usual difficulties still remain about further additions to it by other unknown authors since the time of Nagarjuna. One customary hurdle is that a number of candidates appear at

[88] See note 27 above, p. xxxi.

various time of history with the name of Nagarjuna to add to the confusion and chaos. But the stature of Nagarjuna who was connected to the court of King Kanishka stands out and many opinions completely agree with regard to his contribution to *Susruta Samhita*. The quote below from Meulenbeld is sufficient to cite here in support that Nagarjuna was the first who completely rewrote *Susruta Samhita*.[89]

> Nagarjuna is the first reviser of *Susruta Samhita* and he lived during the reign of Kanishka.

This agreement among a majority of analysts as pointed out above leads us to believe that both the primary medical texts known as *Caraka Samhita* and *Susruta Samhita* were completely re-written about the same times in Gandhara and later Dridabala produced his own additions and commentary of *Caraka Samhita* and at later date Dalhana did the same for *Susruta Samhita*. Nevertheless the above arguments will not end the controversies or help arriving at any decisive conclusion with regard to the origin of these texts and the debate or uncertainties will go on.

Bhela Samhita as pointed earlier is another treatise that was written by one of the six pupils of Atreya. Although there is evidence that this was available till about 4th century CE and authors of *Bower Manuscript* have borrowed three prescriptions from it. But its where about remained unknown till a single manuscript belonging to 9th century CE was discovered in Central Asia. Its Sanskrit grammar is not what linguists will call classical, showing similarity to other texts created and compiled in Gandhara. It is in the form of dialogue between the teacher Atreya and his pupil Bhela. The contents are purely medical without any religious or philosophical deviations. There is enough evidence to consider that it belonged to the School of Taxila. It may also be available to Arab and Persian medical authors such as

[89] See note 14 above, vol. I A, p. 339.

Avicenna and possible date of the manuscript has been allocated 400-750 CE.[90]

The last among the three great texts of Ayurvedic medicine after *Caraka Samhita* and *Susruta Samhita* is known as *Astangasangraha* (also written as *Astanga Samgraha*); the author of this massive tom was Vagbhata. He wrote the great medical compendium, which though derives heavily on previous two texts but it is a coalesced form of all the medical knowledge of the time in one big bundle. In other words it may be said that Vagbhata did not copy but developed and evolved from the learning of the ancients. Its popularity over many centuries had no match, for a long time it overshadowed the compendiums left by the old masters both Caraka and Susruta and it is still used in the Ayurvedic schools of South India. With such immense following over the centuries one would imagine every thing about the author who did not belong to remote antiquity must have been researched and documented and known by now. The reality is far from it, very little is known about Vagbhata and diversity of opinions despite the relatively recent age are numerous and widely at odds.

With so much controversies and bare minimal factual information filtered down the time it is a dispiriting task to make an argument regarding the association of Vagbhata with Gandhara, which was destroyed few centuries before his time. However the evidence of his Buddhist background and faith in the teaching of Buddha has been documented by a number of historians who are confident about the validity of their observations and consider his predilection to Buddhism cannot be in doubt. The likelihood of wanderings of the family of Vagbhata may be surmised by the historical ground realities of 6th to 7th century CE, it was testing time for the Buddhists in Gandhara due to mass persecution by the descendents of the White Huns who were now settled

[90] See note 14 above, vol. II A, pp. 13-24.

and had hegemony over multitudes of city states. The harsh conditions and difficult times for the Buddhists were described by the Chinese traveller, who may be considered as an eye witness (see below). He travelled far and wide only a little later than the time of Vagbhata. During his visit to Taxila in 630 CE he found it desolate and in ruins. He has also recorded that the usual safe heaven of Kashmir where at earlier times persecuted Buddhists had found refuge was by now lost because it was in the hands of king Toramana and his son Mihirakula both were ruthless persecutors of Buddhism.[91]

There is archaeological evidence of many small Buddhist settlements scattered in the present province of Sindh on the banks of the River Indus during 6-7th century CE. These were the refuge for those who were uprooted from Gandhara. The remnants of some of these settlements and Buddhist monasteries and stupas have recently been discovered in Sindh.[92] It is generally agreed that Vagbhata was born in Sindh in the area what is now Karachi in Pakistan, in a family of famous physicians and learned medicine from his father and another teacher who was a Buddhist. We also know the name of his father was Simhagupta or Sanghagupta, which appears at the end of every chapter in his book. The religious persuasion of Vagbhata has been comprehensively discussed by Meulenbeld under a separate heading that ends in the conclusion that Vagbhata was undoubtedly a Buddhist.[93]

> Buddhist elements (in his writings) that can be hardly questioned are, first of all, a series of names known from the Buddhist pantheon.

---

[91] See note 31 above, p. 67.

[92] Khushik QA. 'Remains of Buddhist era await archaeology department's attention', *Dawn,* Karachi: March 22, 2007.

[93] See note 14 above, vol. I A, pp. 602-609.

The implication reached in the above quote is further supported by the very first lines in the opening chapter of *Astangasangraha*.[94]

> Obeisances to the Buddha, who by the power of knowledge and spells has subdued the mighty serpent called the *citta* (mind) whose head is the prolonged, unrealistic and varied kind of desires; whose hood the hatred ness; whose poison is the lust and anger; whose fangs the unreasonable logic; whose frightening eyes the greed; whose face is delusion and who dwells within the crevices of body.

The precise period of Vagbhata has not yet been determined or agreed beyond doubt but majority seem to accept a period during 7th century CE when *Astangasangraha* was compiled. Although sooner we enter this debate we are hampered by the conventional difficulties due to want of information on historical events and poverty in chronology. The difficulties are further multiplied by the fact that there is another text known as *Astangahrydaya* or heart of medicine (also written as *Astanga Hridya*) by Vagbhata. The historians have devised a solution by thinking up or conjuring a convenient solution that there were two different persons that existed, one was Vagbhata I or senior and other was Vagbhata II or junior. Added to this is another speculation that the two Vagbhatas were a team of father and son. Still no hard evidence can be put forward about who wrote what but arbitrarily the *Astangasangraha* has been allocated to the senior or the father and *Astangahrydaya* to the junior or the son. A third opinion that both the texts were written by one Vagbhata is also not beyond the realm of possibilities. The *Astangasangraha* is larger containing far more details; it can be compared to a reference book while *Astangahrydaya* is a kind of shorter version or concise edition much suited as a text book for the students. The Arab physicians of 8th and 9th century CE have quoted from the *Astangasangraha* and it is

---

[94] Murthy KRS, tr., *Astangasamargraha*, Varanasi: Chowkambha Orientalia, 1995, p. 1.

also mentioned that it was translated into Persian or Arabic, but no such manuscript has ever come to light. Since the *Astangasangraha* remained available and accessible right from its earliest times, there are hardly any commentaries on it. The only commentary is said to be written by a person only known by the name of Indu and most probably lived about 10th century CE.

A comparative analysis and critical study of the three medical compendia together with the *Bower Manuscript* no doubt would be an extremely worthwhile, but unfortunately such an exercise has never been under taken. Even a cursory look in a systematic fashion at all the four texts may bring out many features that are common. The surgery in Vagbhata is almost similar to what we see in *Susruta Samhita,* for example the details of the surgical instruments and their names are identical. The aphorism that the best surgical instrument is the hand (or fingers) of a skilful surgeon is virtually repeated verbatim. But some of the operative procedures in Vagbhata have somewhat more details. This can be illustrated from the account of the operation that may be described a post-mortem caesarean section recommended when the mother has died at full term and the movements of the foetus are observed. In such a circumstance in order to save the unborn an immediate operation is strongly advised both by Susruta and Vagbhata. But only Vagbhata has elaborated further by explaining that the site of the incision must be over the region of the bladder. It is obvious that Vagbhata was deeply inspired and heavily relied on both Caraka and Susruta to which he added his own reflections. As a result he was able to compile a better and more practicable text that remained a medical guide for a long time over shadowing the two original ancient works. Nevertheless the wisdom contained in Vagbhata may be widely taught and applied for a number of centuries; there is no evidence that during the centuries before, during or after Vagbhata, the surgery was ever practised by professional surgeons in a rational fashion. Despite Vagbhata's dispensing of older medicine in new jazzed up bottles the decline in Indian surgery that was set at the time of the destructions of Buddhist Monasteries continued never to revive again. It seems obvious that the decline in surgery is closely linked to the banishment of Buddhism. In other words with Buddhism the surgery was also exiled and the indications are that Ayurvedic Medicine had migrated to the monasteries in the land of China adjoining with Gandhara. This conclusion we can derive from the very fact that the *Bower Manuscript* was discovered in a Chinese monastery, but it is also noticeable that apparently surgery did not blossom even there.

All the above four texts in their methodology are broadly treatment centric of the conditions diagnosed on the basis of symptoms and it will be worth while to see how they come up to treat a given symptom. If we chose cough that is labelled *Kasa* by all the four texts and then see how they dealt, it might be worthwhile exercise.

The *Caraka Samhita* starts the section on the treatment of cough with the following sentence.

> We shall expound the treatment of cough, thus said the illustrious one of Atri's race.

Then the text fills nearly twenty five pages dealing with a variety of coughs and many formulae or prescriptions are recorded to treat the cough. The methods of treatments cover huge range from local applications to inhalations and medicines to be taken by mouth, clarified butter or Ghee with honey comes quite often in to discussion.

In the *Susruta Samhita* the cough or *Kasa* is included in the final chapter that is generally regarded to be wholly an addition by Dridabala. It approaches the subject more methodically, enumerating firstly the causes then a discussion about five different types and still longer discourse on symptoms. In the treatment a number of foods prepared with specific ingredients are mentioned, concentrated juice of sugar cane after cooking, honey and clarified butter are mentioned here too. Inhalations are also mentioned but not elaborated a great deal.

Vagbhata in his *Astangasangraha* starts the chapter with 'thus said Atreya and other sages', which follows many pages of discussion. The essential underline emphasis is very similar as described by the previous two texts and not much new material can be identified, which is expected because it was the last to be written after fairly long intervening period, condensing the material found in the earlier books. The use of clarified butter and honey is common with others as mentioned before.

The chapter on treatment of cough in the *Bower Manuscript* is not as methodical as in others. It is not consolidated under one heading but scattered all over the text. The basic style is similar where many formulae are mentioned, the clarified butter, honey and use of inhalations are also recorded.

This brief comparison of the treatment of cough in all four texts typifies the essence and core of the subject matter and shows that the approach to various topics is not greatly far removed from each other. On the other hand it is also hard to establish with certainty that the later writers copied from their forerunners. Although it is obvious that the succeeding authors or compilers had a strong sense of dedicated loyalty to the old masters and seem to stand in awe in the reverence of their predecessors. They followed the *gurus* devotedly and did not divert from the style and ideology of the ancients. To allude to the example of Galen and later of Avicenna may be proper and appropriate; in both cases for centuries any opinion conflicting with their teachings was considered a sin equivalent to heresy. Such steadfast adherence always discouraged new thinking and progress and ultimately resulting in stagnation. This situation prevailed far longer in the Ayurvedic dogma, as a result through a long period of the history Ayurvedic Medicine remained bogged down in rituals and stifled without any evolution of new ideas ever taking place. In other words concepts remained static because same ideas kept on repeating themselves again and again. The contents of all the major works despite many centuries apart show no evolving process. Probably the only exception is the first chapter on garlic in the *Bower Manuscript* a one rare example of new way of thinking.

Nevertheless a complete analysis regarding the poverty of new ideas with in the texts discussed above is not easy. Such a study requires the application of modern methodologies using present day computers and pertinent software that would provide some logical way for a comparative and critical analysis of these texts. Some of these methods have been talk about and discussed by the historiographers.[95] More advance current methods might also solve the difficulties of chronology and some other on going controversies. Without such sophisticated methods we can only infrequently observe evidence of inherent replication in some areas as pointed out here in the few examples.

The manner of invoking the blessing of the ultimate teachers in the beginning and at the end of each chapter is uniformly employed in all the above texts.

As for as therapeutics is concerned all the four texts have many treatments that are common and the constituents of the prescriptions recorded in them remain similar; while in some cases exactly the same. The obstetrics and gynaecology in the three compendiums remained unaltered while the *Bower Manuscript* contains no surgery at all.

---

[95] Clarke E. ed., *Modern methods in the history of medicine*, London: The Athlon Press, 197, pp. 195-211.

The pathology based on the imbalance of the humours that is the basis of the causes of all diseases remains same and virtually unchanged in all the texts and the principle to reverse this imbalance also continued as the key to treatments. Such standard believes had been repeated one after the other for centuries without any attempt to entertain any other ideology or doctrine.

The standard of anatomy and physiology does not show any evolutionary progress even with the passing of many centuries. There are some differences in the total number of bones in the human body. The *Susruta Samhita* tells us the total number of bones is 300 and that the earlier writers have mentioned the number 360. One such text that gives this number is *Caraka Samhita;* that clearly puts *Caraka Samhita* anterior to *Susruta Samhita.*

The *Caraka Samhita* and the *Bower Manuscript* both deal mostly with internal medicine where surgery is only mentioned in passing, while the surgery and the surgical instruments in other two works are practically similar though the stated intervening period might be more than half a millennium.

All the four texts discussed in the above paragraphs have one important common feature, they have not utilised any diagnostic techniques and not mentioned the pulse at all. Jolly in his assessment of the ancient Indian medical texts has pointed out that in Indian medical literature absence of the mention of the pulse in a text is an evidence of its antiquity.[96]

When compared with the contemporary Greek and Roman texts like *De Medicina* of Celsus, writings of Galen and Soranus, it becomes obvious that the three major Indian medical texts lack the rational approach in almost all areas.

---

[96] Jolly J. *Indian Medicine,* tr., Kashikar CG, New Delhi: Munshiram Manoharlal Publishers, 1977, p.12.

The lack of the pulse examination for diagnostic purposes as pointed out above also put them lesser to the Chinese and Greek system of medicine of comparable periods.

The notable drawback or disadvantage due to total lack of any influence from other sources, the Sanskrit medical texts seem to have suffered, was yet another reason that resulted in seriously restricting the progress. It is fair observation and the events of history vouch that exchange between civilisations as a result of interaction of knowledge brings about freshness in thinking. The fact that up till tenth century CE Sanskrit literature including medical literature remained without any influence from out side, as a result there was a massive stagnation. The absence of exchange that should have resulted in evolutionary progress of ideas caused a kind of isolation, a fact most noticeable in medical texts. The Sanskrit texts over the centuries remained almost rigidly obdurate, replicating the same thoughts again and again. It is further surprising that the opportunities of interchange with other civilisations were available but due to unexplained reasons failed to materialise or make any impact. There were thriving contacts over many centuries with China through a number of travellers and via trade connections with the Romans and direct interactions with the Greek through conquests. All these prolonged exchanges had little influence on the Sanskrit literature and none at all on the medical literature in any way. There is no evidence that any medical text from out side was ever translated into Sanskrit. On the other hand visitors from outside such as Chinese, Persians, and Arabs and later the Western scholars made good use from what they could learn from the translations they carried out from the Sanskrit texts and enriched their literature.

8.
The Chinese Buddhist pilgrims in Gandhara

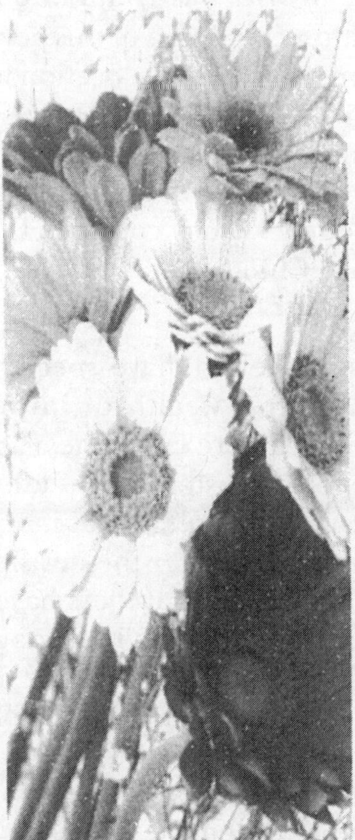

Once the Buddhism took firm roots in China a number of Buddhist monks travelled to India as pilgrims visiting the sacred Buddhist centres and also to seek out the scriptures. They must have valued Gandhara highly consecrated because most if not all seem to have visited the sacred Buddhist sites at remote corners all over Gandhara. These were scattered at great distances and their access through the highest mountains in the World was tremendously challenging. However the Buddhist Gandhara of this period due to charity of the people was most hospitable location for any peripatetic traveller in the attire of a holy man. He was assured a decent sustenance, accommodation and safety just by knocking any door during his wonderings. Begging for food was a kind of veneration and people would consider themselves blessed if a holy man from China comes to their door asking for food, shelter and protection.

Three of these travellers have special place in history because they have left a wealth of information in their accounts. Their records were eye witness accounts that carry great significance to the history of Buddhism in Gandhara because their visits happened to be at intervals of roughly a century before, during and after the invasion of White Hun. The names of these Chinese travellers have cropped up few times at linked topics in previous pages, but a brief chronological depiction of their travels at this stage is highly relevant, which should be pertinent and helpful. Aurel Stein who visited most of the sites that have been described by the three most important Chinese travellers has repetitively pointed out and underlined the places and the legends in relation to these places as described by his forerunners. In order to fully understand in current context the places mentioned in the accounts of Fa Hien, Sung Yun and Hsuan Tsang the reports of Aurel Stein about ancient Khotan is an essential reading.[97] The Chinese travellers though travelled all over India spending long period of time at many sacred Buddhists monasteries, here the discussion will confine to their wonderings in Gandhara only.

Fa Hien who travelled from central China to Gandhara was among the many pilgrims who took this route before and after him but he must be considered the first who lived long enough to record a comprehensive travel log on reaching back in China. The period of his travels commencing in about 399 CE and ended in 412 CE when he returned back to his homeland. These dates have been suggested by the analysts who have studied his works and the fact that he has recorded the events of Gupta dynasty of the time. He followed the Silk Road from Western China and has documented some of the names of places in the inaccessible mountains passes that can be recognised even today. At the time of his visit Buddhism as well as Gandhara art had reached the peak and his eye witness accounts of the splendour of the Buddhist cities is vividly reflected in his narrative.[98] The records left by Fa Hien also corroborate many historical aspects related to Buddhist sacred locations, the relics placed in them and rituals linked with the sacred objects. A number of the objects discovered in archaeological excavations at various places in Gandhara were seen and visited by Fa Hien during his travels. The shrines where the sanctified relics of Buddha's bone and tooth were discovered after one and a half millennium were clearly identified by him. Through out Gandhara he found the Buddhism was flourishing noting its strong influence on political, social and

---

[97] Stein MA. *Ancient Khotan. Detailed report of archaeological explorations in Chinese Turkistan*, Oxford: The Clarendon Press, 1907. Full text and photographs of all the pages available free at, http://dsr.nii.ac.jp/toyobunko/VIII-5B2-7/V/page/0005.html.en.

[98] See note 57 above.

cultural activities of the people who were prosperous and living in peace. Most of the stupas he has described were decorated with plates of gold and silver, while the kings and rulers were charitable, enthusiastically engaged in religious rites. The glimpses about the social structure and functioning of society in Gandhara, which Fa Hien has described makes valuable records to understand the history of a period that was later, clouded in uncertainties. Although he has not provided us with any direct information or detailed information on medical care but he specifically noted that the offerings from pious citizens were used to maintain places from where all sort of care was provided to the devotees. His further remark about the peace and safety is also noteworthy that according to him was prevalent every where. In his search of Buddhist scriptures he travelled from Gandhara to Ceylon or present day Sri Lanka from where he took the hazardous sea route back to China and passed rest of his life in meditating, writing and translating the *Vinaya Patika* into Chinese, which is still used by the Buddhist monasteries in China, Japan and Korea as a code of discipline. It also contains guidance for the Monks on healthy living, nursing care of the sick and rudimentary medicine applied to the Buddhist monastic life. The care of the sick within the monasteries as alluded to above, in fact was a legacy from Buddha himself, which according to Buddhist traditions had ordered to all his followers during the early stages of the campaign of the new faith.

Sung Yun was the second notable Chinese Buddhist pilgrim who visited Gandhara between 518 to 521 CE. It is recorded by his biographer that he was sponsored by the Empress of China to travel the West from where he had to seek out and bring back the genuine Buddhist scriptures from the Buddhist monasteries. He travelled west along the Silk Road and then south into present Afghanistan to reach Gandhara. Most significant aspect of his account is the narrative about the control of Gandhara by the White Huns and though the White Huns were tormenters of the

Buddhist faith the Buddhism was not yet completely banished from Gandhara at the time of the visit by Sung Yun. His homewards journey was the way he came. Unfortunately no original records of his written accounts have survived; whatever is available today is what others have quoted long after his death. His sole interest was in the scriptures and spiritual interaction with the monks of famous monasteries. He made no observations regarding social aspects of the people living in Gandhara and has not offered any opinion on medical texts or the medical care or practice of surgery in Gandhara during the early 6th century CE. Some woolly stories are associated with his records but these might have been supplemented by later sources to make the tale more action-packed or beguiling to the audience or sponsors. One such story is about the elephants trained for warfare with swords fastened to their trunks thus creating havoc among the enemies of Huna.[99]

The last of the three and the most celebrated Chinese traveller who visited Gandhara was Hsuan Tsang (599-664 CE). He started his journey from Xian that was capital of China, probably in 629 CE and returned after seventeen years of travelling throughout Gandhara and other Buddhist sites all over India. From China he travelled further west along the Silk Road up to Samarqand and then south to present Afghanistan, from where he entered into Gandhara crossing the Khyber Pass. His must be the most fulfilling life because he was successful in achieving all his aims that he had set for himself before the journey, 'to visit the holy places, to see the shrines, to study scriptures in original language and bring back the Buddhist scriptures from the Buddhist monasteries'. He had adopted monastic life at a very young age and was fully ordained a monk in 622 CE but was not happy when he discovered enormous discrepancies in the Buddhist texts available in China. This prompted him first to master Sanskrit and other languages to study the scriptures

[99] See note 31 above, p.129.

in original languages and then embarked on the long journey of self education. Although in the writings linked to Hsuan Tsang there is no mention about the medical or surgical conventions in those areas he visited, but his observations regarding the customs and social lives of the people of Gandhara are highly significant being the eye witness accounts at the time when Buddhism was declining in Gandhara. He has made passing comments regarding the teaching of Ayurveda while discussing the education and other learning. These comments of Hsuan Tsang were in connection with the school of Nalanda where he stayed quite few years learning the scriptures. His minimal interest in matters of medical teaching or practice is understandable since his primary interest lay in the Buddhist scriptures and he himself was not a medical person. This is unlike yet another well known Chinese visitor; I tsing who travelled to India only a short period after Hsuan Tsang. I tsing himself practised medicine and also wrote about monastic medical practices but never visited the North or Gandhara at all.

Hsuan Tsang had visited almost all known Buddhist sites in Gandhara, including many of those which are remote and extremely difficult to access even today. After visiting the two famous giant Buddhas at Bamyan (now destroyed) and other monasteries on the way he must have walked through the Khyber Pass to reach what he described Kanishka's Vihara in the city he called as Pulushapulu or Pushpapura, now known as Peshawar. His detailed and accurate description of the size and height of this grand stupa being the largest and tallest any where; provided not only inspiration but also helped in locating and then excavating it in 1908.[100] In the accounts of Hsuan-Tsang we also discover interesting comments recorded about the social life of the people living in this area. He noted giving details that he found the people were markedly different in manners, clothing and language than other places he had

[100] See note 32 above, p.138.

visited. He reached Taxila in about 631 CE and found it in ruin and the city was under the firm control of the kingdom of Kashmir governed by the Huns. Else where in Gandhara he found few monasteries that were saved from the Hun destruction where Mahayana Buddhism was practiced. He himself became a student of Mahayana School and studied under a learned monk staying in a remote monastery in Kashmir. He then travelled up to Lumbini, the birth place of Buddha; visited and wrote about the pillar which Ashoka had erected at the site.

When Hsuan Tsang returned home he brought with him over 600 Sanskrit books of Buddhist canon, settling down in a monastery out side the capital Xian to translate the Sanskrit scriptures in to the local language. This ancient monastery is now known as Da Cien Temple and is also the home of the famous seven story high Big Wild Goose Pagoda. At this pleasant place he spent another seventeen years in translating the books he had brought and also writing his travel log. The Temple holds many of the relics that were brought by Hsuan Tsang back from his travels. A huge statue of Hsuan Tsang is prominently standing in the square of the temple with Big Wild Goose Pagoda in the back ground (Fig.13). It is probably the most photographed panorama in the old capital of China today. Hsuan Tsang died in 664 CE.

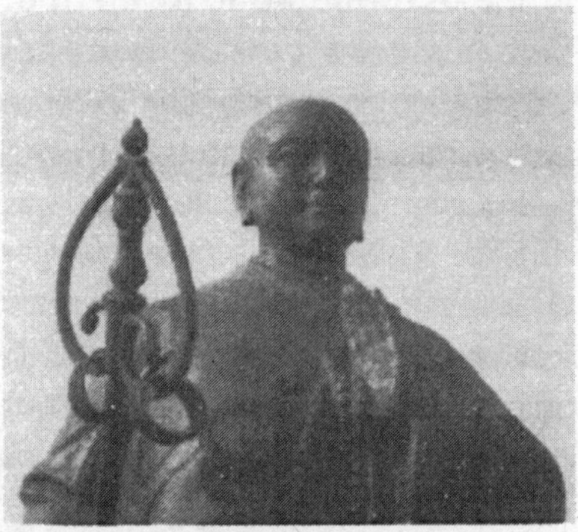

Fig. 13

Statue of Hsuan Tsang at the Pagoda of Great Wild Goose, Xian, China.

As for as link between Gandhara and Tibetan Buddhism and Tibetan medicine is concerned it is difficult to trace any association during the early period but the Chinese Buddhist contacts with Tibet were well established later through the Silk Road. The evidence may be seen in the manuscripts of Buddhist canon that were discovered during late nineteenth century in Tibet. One of these is known as *Dutreuil de Rhins Manuscript* (after the French man who discovered it). It was part of Buddhist sacred text, most probably written in Gandhari.

As for as Tibetan medicine is concerned it strongly remained shamanic for a long period; later only very slowly was influenced by the Chinese medicine. There is sufficient evidence of any external influence due to the isolation of the territory, but as late as the seventh century CE some evidence of Buddhist medical influence is noticeable due to Buddhist monks from China. This seems to have more potent effect when the king of Tibet was converted to Buddhism and ordered the books on Buddhist scriptures and Ayurvedic Medicine to be brought from India. This is how the Vagbhata's Astangasangraha found its way in to Tibet. The Tibetan Medicine had retained some of the shamanic originality along with the Chinese Medicine and later by Ayurvedic Medicine. This is probably how the Tibetan Medicine developed its own unique form. In the West during recent times there has been greater awareness as regard to the Tibetan Medicine, particularly the Tibetan surgery; that has survived almost intact from the ancient times. But no archaeologically excavated ancient surgical instruments have ever come to light. Although some pictures of Tibetan surgical instruments on a chart are sold in antique markets of India, China and Tibet and on the internet. The instruments illustrated in these pictures have no archaeological validation and carry no similarity with the known Buddhist excavated surgical instruments discovered in Gandhara. Moreover the historical events tell us that before the Ayurvedic medicine reached Tibet the surgery had long died even in India. But the influence of Chinese Medicine on Tibetan medicine using the pulse in diagnosis, massage and acupuncture remained more dominating than the medicine of Caraka and Susruta and Vagbhata that was imported from India.

In summary from the available information we can gather it is obvious that as for as the Tibetan medicine is concerned there were contacts with China through which the Buddhist Canon and medical texts reached Tibet. This exchange must have included the Buddhist scripture, medical and other material that had travelled from Gandhara to China. But at a much later stage Buddhist Medical texts were imported into Tibet from India, though the Tibetan medicine has retained some of its old and original shaman characters.

9.
Medical archaeology of Gandhara

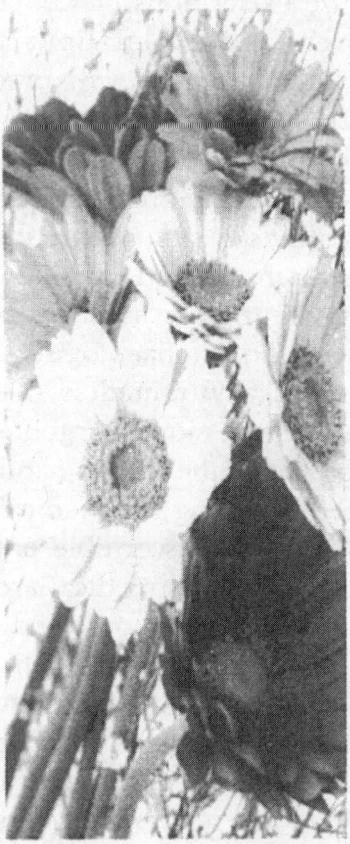

Medical archaeology although a relatively young speciality, even then it is now a well defined and established discipline that has evolved through history of medicine, medical anthropology and archaeology. It is also true to a large extent that the medical archaeology was a spin off from the study of surgical instruments that were discovered in huge numbers from the excavations of Roman and Greek sites. After the discovery and explorations of Pompeii, where largest hoards of extremely well made and preserved medical artefacts and surgical instruments were found. These remained buried under the ash not cnly in large numbers but also protected from elements such as wet and damp soil. These finds created tremendous interest among the archaeologists, who started to document and catalogue these surgical instruments as early as first half of the nineteenth century. The archaeologists who had discovered them were not medically trained so they have to seek the help or opinion of professional surgeons, obstetricians and gynaecologists to explain the working and uses of these finds. This created interest among the medical fraternity some of them were involved with discernible enthusiasm and were probably wrongly labelled as medical archaeologists. At the same time the contributions of some of these earliest medical men interested in archaeology were valuable and are widely quoted as reliable works of reference. The co-operation that flourished among the medically trained individuals and professional archaeologists was successful and had proved to be fruitful. Nonetheless over the years the developments in osteo-archaeology and the increasing influence of academic social historians helped to widen the medical archaeology into a separate and broader discipline. As a result its area of interest has grown far beyond the limitations of merely recognising the unusual, rusty metal pieces that in the remote past might have been used as surgical instruments. At present the study of excavated artefacts or surgical instruments from which the medical archaeology had come into being, is only a small part of medical archaeology. An all-encompassing history of medical archaeology is yet to be compiled that might illustrate the essential changes that have influenced the aims and methodologies from the time of Karl Sudhoff (1853-1938) who was the first to establish the medical archaeology and laid down the methodology and objectives in 1926.[101]

The social archaeology of Gandhara is obviously not relevant and out of the scope of the forthcoming discussion where it is indented to review the artefacts excavated in Gandhara that are related to medicine or appear to be surgical instruments and ascertain their uses by comparing them with similar known objects of analogous period excavated from Greek or Roman sites. In previous pages at appropriate places mere reference to such archaeological finds had been alluded to, but the ensuing discussion is essentially to examine in greater details the medical artefacts or surgical instruments that were excavated over a long period of time at various sites in Gandhara.

When we look or search the literature with regard to excavated surgical instruments, it becomes clear that no such objects have ever been discovered any where in the World except in Greek or in the lands which had been under the influence of Romans. Among the other ancient civilisations of corresponding periods though historical evidence of surgery of capricious veracity is forthcoming but it is not collaborated with archaeological evidence. In other words

---

[101] Sudhoff K. 'Aims, means and methods in medical archaeology,' Alleman A. tr. *Essays in the history of medicine*, New York: Medical life Press, 1926, pp. 157-58.

till now there was almost total lack of archaeological surgical instruments among all other cultures except Greek and Romans. Such a notion might be surprising but it is a fact that cannot be disproved. It is worthwhile to mention about a hoard of about fifty surgical instruments excavated in old Cairo at the site known as Al Fustat. These were discovered at an unknown date and claimed to be from late Umayyad or early Abbasid period (approximately 740-800 CE).[102] Unfortunately the referred paper has not indicated where these objects are displayed and no mention is made if any archaeological assessment has ever been carried out. More importantly no attempt is made to judge their date either from the layers they were found or by other scientific dating methods available today. In the absence of necessary required technical data this hoard apparently of genuine surgical instruments consisting probes, cauteries, knives, spatulas, a pair of scissors, needles etc may belong to Greek, Roman, Byzantine or possibly Arabic period.

The Buddhist medicine and surgery has never been independently discussed by the medical historians but remains part of Indian medicine and surgery, which of course is a subject that has been copiously written about. All scholarly texts or opinions on the topic of surgery in India have unanimous agreement that surgical instruments have never been discovered in any archaeological excavations any where to corroborate the historical data in respect of surgery. In support of this premise citing of few of the germane references and quotes from acknowledged sources is of paramount importance.

A number of modern publications on Indian medicine including few of the translations of *Susruta Samhita* contain diagrams of surgical instruments which in reality have been based on pure fantasy but presented as authentic Susrutan

[102] Hamarneh SK, Awad HA. 'Early surgical instruments excavated in old Cairo, Egypt' in *International Surgery*, 1977; 62: pp. 520-24.

instruments. In fact there is no tradition of diagrammatic expressions in the ancient Indian medical writings or even those from the Middle Ages, such an opinion has been documented in recent publications.[103]

All the surgical instruments that have been illustrated in these publications claim to be the authentic historical instruments. But none offers the ultimate source of these imaginary drawings. But the earliest source of these drawings can be traced to three nineteenth century publications from where all others have copied the drawings without citing the original publications. The first was published by T. A. Wise in 1845 which illustrated 24 surgical instruments where as the drawings are of high professional quality but not based on any real objects, rather all are inventive and hypothetically created after the designs of ubiquitous surgical instruments of the time.[104] The second was published in 1879 in Bengali language by Kaviraj Binod Lal Sen titled *Ayurveda Vijnana.* This was a kind of summary of all the Sanskrit medical texts available to the author and contained diagrams of the surgical instruments supposedly as described in some of the texts.[105] The third source was a paper in the journal of the Buddhist Text Society of India published in 1894, listing nearly one hundred diagrams of surgical instruments. It also contained yet more drawings of the Tibetan surgical instruments as well. From these three original publications the diagrams of surgical instruments were copied and some were modified by H.H. Bhagvat Sinh Jee in his publication of 1896.[106] (This publication is presently available under four

[103] Wujastyk D. 'A Persian anatomical image in a non-Muslim manuscript from Gujarat,' in *Medical History,* 2007, pp. 237-42.

[104] Wise TA. *Commentary on the Hindu system of medicine,* Calcutta: the Baptist Mission Press, 1845.

[105] Das K. *Obstetric forceps: its history and evolution,* Leeds: Medical Museum, 1993 (First edition 1929).

[106] Bhagvat Sinh Jee HH. *A short history of Aryan medical science,* London: Macmillan and Co. Ltd., 1896.

different titles by four different publishers) It contained pictures from Wise and about 64 other drawings of surgical instruments claimed to be after the description from Susruta. In this publication there are diagrams of many pharmaceutical implements as well. Most of these were then copied in a much cited publication from 1910 titled, *'The surgical instruments of the Hindus'*. Only the last author has acknowledged the fact that no surgical instruments of Indian origin have ever been excavated and the drawings were merely imaginary. Many of the drawings in size, shape and general construction are apparently based on the dental forceps of the period and it is clear that no professional surgeon was ever consulted because the designs of the instruments depicted in the diagrams would be of little use in practical surgery. More importantly the author while discussing the excavated surgical instruments from Greek and Roman sites and exhibited in the museums of Athens, Naples and other European cities made the following comment.[107]

> But as far as I have been able to trace, our museums contain no finds supplying us with any information on the subject.

Further down few pages in the preface he has also unambiguously stated as quoted below that all such drawings of the instruments in his monograph were imaginary representations, although this fact has been totally ignored by many of those who reproduced the same drawings as genuine instruments.

> To complete the subject, I have added plates of nearly all the varieties of instruments; but they are more or less hypothetical as we do not possess any actual specimens of the instruments of Hindus.

---

[107] Mukhopadhyaya G. *The surgical instruments of the Hindus, with a comparative study of surgical instruments of the Greek, Roman, Arab and the modern European surgeon,* New Delhi: R.K. Nahar and Co., reprint 1977, (First published 1909) pp. iv, xii.

This well known text published almost a century ago is excellent for the historical commentary but when comes to make a comparison of surgical instruments with Greek, Roman, Arab and modern instruments, an objective stated in its title, it unfortunately put up a disappointing performance. Nearly half the pages of the book contain unrelated pictures from 1895-1903 catalogues of the British surgical instruments makers like Arnold and Sons, Allen and Hanburys and pictures from the texts of surgery of the period. The pictures from these sources of surgical instruments and other appliances are interspersed with the imaginary drawings while the text singularly fails to make a comparative study with Greek, Roman or any Arab instruments.

Another highly referred and esteemed publication recommended as a text book for the students of history of medicine has also touched this issue implying that no surgical instruments have ever been discovered from any Indian archaeological site.[108]

> Medical texts do not contain any development of surgical ideas, nor do any genuinely ancient or medieval surgical instruments survive. Surgery is not described in literary or other sources... .

In order to search for ancient surgical instruments in the museums the author has visited and enquired at the National Museum of India in Delhi, Lahore Museum and Peshawar Museum in Pakistan but has not been able to locate any exhibits that might have suggestion of a surgical instrument used in ancient times. Similarly inquiries by letters from other major museums in India such as Kolkata, Chennai and Allahabad, which otherwise hold many other objects excavated in Gandhara have also resulted in negative. These museums do not hold any artefacts or proper surgical instruments. On personal inquiry (January 2002) to Mr.

---

[108] Bynum WF, Potter R. eds., *Companion Encyclopaedia of history of medicine*, vol. I, London: Routledge, 1993, p. 763.

Ralph Jackson, curator of the Romano-British collection at British Museum, London, information was provided that no surgical instruments of Indian or Buddhist origin exist at the British Museum either. This pretty much covers all those museums where the relevant artefacts might have been stored or exhibited but it is evident such objects do not exist at these museums. The only museum where the surgical instruments are exhibited is the Taxila museum and these exhibits are to be discussed in detail forthcoming pages.

Furthermore it is also a valid notion that a search should be made into the archaeological catalogues of the famous Buddhist sites which are historically associated with Buddhism and in modern times have been subjected to extensive archaeological investigations over a long period of time. It is likely that excavations at these sites may have brought to light the surgical instruments that might have been used in the monasteries where surgical treatment was offered by the Buddhist Monks.

One such site of great historical importance is Pataliputra, which has been and still is an exalted centre not only for Buddhism but Hinduism as well. This famous centre came in the limelight from about the time of Buddha as it is not mentioned in the early Vedas and Sanskrit epic literature. The ancient locations around this sacred site have been surveyed and excavations were carried out for many years. During 1955-1956 it was subjected to extensive archaeological activity targeting the places that were proven monasteries. The result of this activity was published in 1970.[109] The catalogue has listed masses of metal objects of iron as well as copper but no surgical instruments have been listed and neither any comment are recorded by the authors as regard to their absence.

---

[109] Sinha BP, Narain LA. *Pataliputra excavations 1955-56,* Patna: The Directorate of archaeology and museums, Patna, 1970.

Another well established and sacred place mentioned in the texts from ancient times is Visali. Its association with Buddhism is also proven, in Jataka literature it gets mentioned on numerous occasions. Here excavations were carried out from 1958-1962 followed by the publication of the investigations in 1969.[110] The search of this publication also proved negative as for as any surgical instruments or similar implements are concerned, although as usual many other metal objects are listed in huge numbers.

The third important archaeological site included in the search was Kapilvastu, its significance being the birth place of the Buddha cannot be emphasised more by using any superlatives. Although a purely archaeological survey of Kapilvastu was not available, instead a historical text was consulted which included fair amount of archaeological information as well.[111] Once more no trace or even a mere mention as regard any kind of surgical instruments or related material was forthcoming.

It is important to mention that one reason put forward for the near total lack of the excavated surgical instruments from ancient Indian archaeological sites is that the damp climate due to heavy monsoon and then intense heat during summer perished the metal objects buried under the damp soil leaving no trace. At the same times further argument is made that the reason surgical instruments of Roman origin were buried under the ash and remained well preserved, while such objects did not survive in the damp soil in India. This is not at all a valid explanation because all museums exhibit thousands of other metal objects of all sizes in fairly reasonable state of preservation. The logic and common sense dictates that the reasons for the absence of medical related objects or actual surgical instruments must be some

---

[110] Sinha BP, Roy SR. *Visali excavations 1958-1962,* Patna: Directorate of archaeology and museums, Patna, 1969.

[111] Srivastava KM. *Discovery of Kapilvastu,* New Delhi: Books and Books, 1986.

where else. A credible or likely explanation might be that somehow such objects have not yet been found at many sites. But at least at some sites within Gandhara the archaeologists had a lucky turn where a number of genuine tools of surgery were excavated. One such site is Taxila, a place well known for its medical education.

The most recent surgical implement in Gandhara was excavated during late 2007 at a newly discovered site about ten kilometres north-east of Taxila. It is too early to have full archaeological appraisal or complete details regarding the nature, period and utility of this newly discovered surgical instrument. Its discovery was announced along with few other valuable objects such as a gold coin of early Kushan period.

This fresh archaeological discovery of an object related to surgery more than seventy years after the last finds in Taxila is immensely noteworthy, it reiterates and supports the view that all what is buried under the earth is yet to be unearthed. Moreover Gandhara is the only place which has revealed at more than one site the surgical instruments or related objects that can be compared with Greek and Roman excavated instruments, again a hugely significant fact. These discoveries at historically known seat of medical education during the period of Buddhist pre-eminence, offer undeniable validation of surgical practice in this region.

It is also important to look into the sources of metal ore, mining and metallurgical skills of the people of Gandhara who designed and made those instruments that will be discussed shortly. All civilisations emerging from Stone Age have exploited metals, creating a variety of tools and particularly weapons to kill for foods or fight with enemies. It is recorded that man obtained copper by smelting even before he discovered iron. There is well founded archaeological evidence of smelting copper and iron in Mesopotamia during the seventh millennium BCE. These two metals were also widely used from the time of Harappan civilisation, from where a number of copper seals and many other metal objects have been excavated.[112] In Gandhara and its neighbourhood both these metals were mined but the deposits were not huge. There is some indication that the copper might have been imported from other places. Although the discovery of metal objects from remote antiquity going back to Vedic period is not forthcoming but the quality of metal and skill of manufacturing from the iron pillars that are still standing offers a convincing evidence for the expertise of metal workers of the period. A number of inscriptions on silver and copper that were discovered in Taxila also provide a strong indication as regard to the use of different metals in a variety of uses.[113] This is further reinforced from the quantity of iron and copper objects seen in the museums offering adequate confirmation that these metals were abundantly available and the artisans had reached a high level of metallurgical skills, a fact which can be observed uniformly through out ancient Gandhara.

The surgical instruments to be discussed belong to a period extending to last couple of centuries of last millennium BCE and about first two centuries of the first millennium CE. The examples of art or utility objects from the same period that can be seen exhibited in the museums within Gandhara allow no misgiving about the expertise in designing and manufacturing quality objects. The metal workers were perfectly capable to create and tailor-make tools of surgery at the order of the surgeons who wanted to use them. This is obvious from the design of spatula made of beaten copper and carry typical Buddhist icon at the end of its handle, which has been described as *'nandipada'*. It

---

[112] Agrawal DP, Ghosh A. eds., 1971, *The Copper-Bronze Age in India,* New Delhi: Munshiram Manoharlal, 1971.

[113] Chanda P. 'Taxila inscription of the year 136.' *The Journal of the Royal Asiatic Society,* July 1920, pp. 319-24. Also see, Deb HK. 'Taxila silver inscription', *The Journal of the Royal Asiatic Society,* January 1922, pp. 37-42.

shows for sure that the objects were locally made. Moreover their manufacturing process seems to be similar to the numerous other metal objects discovered for domestic or trade use. In other words when on the count of design they are compared with Greek and Roman instruments the Gandhara surgical instruments are not copies but stand out as independently designed and crafted in Gandhara.

Another rather important aspect for making a comparison of the Gandhara instruments with majority of Greek and Roman surgical instruments is the selection of metal. The Buddhist instruments found in Gandhara are all made of almost pure copper. In the absence of any other archaeological discoveries of such items made of any other metal it is difficult for us to imagine the reasons or benefits of choosing copper for making surgical instruments and reasons of preference from one metal than other by the makers. Perhaps their predilection to use copper might be due to its property of not rusting as much opposed to iron and thus less chance of decaying. But most probably the choice of copper for making these instruments by the metal workers of Gandhara was its availability and their confidence due to prolonged experience working with their favourite metal. This is obvious from huge number of copper objects that have been discovered in Gandhara. The use of pure copper also makes the distinction from Greek and Roman instruments that Gandhara instruments were designed and manufactured without the influence from out side.

In contrast the Greek traditionally preferred bronze, which contains about 5-10% tin and rest copper. The bronze was not only used in manufacturing the surgical instruments or other medical artefacts but also the objects of art and utensils of daily use. The use of bronze as a proffered metal to make surgical instruments goes back to before the time of Hippocrates. It was natural for Romans to adopt the Greek tradition to use bronze in making the precision instrumentation. The copper was abundantly available with in the Roman Empire; it was extensively mined in Cyprus, Spain and the North African territories of Roman Empire. The Roman instruments of pure copper that have been discovered are only few where as those made of bronze have been found in huge numbers in all parts of the vast Roman Empire. The archaeological finds from Pompeii and Herculaneum, the two major cities that were destroyed in 79 CE and buried under the ash of Vesuvius explosion are of great interest due to their better preservation because they were made of bronze. The Romans also used iron to make instruments, especially those which required sharp edges for cutting such as scalpels or knives. They also designed instruments where cutting edge was made of iron but the handle was of bronze.

On the whole after a detailed comparative analysis an obvious fact comes out in the open that during similar ages the Greek and Roman instruments makers using bronze were able to create more complex and far better quality surgical implements than their opposite numbers in Gandhara. The Gandhara instruments are of simple straight forwards single piece designs except for a pair of forceps. In Gandhara no instruments have been discovered that can match the complexity of Roman instruments, having a controlled mechanism such as opening and closing of the vaginal speculums or others that can be assembled using a number of components. Although in Gandhara a pair of scissors, grasping tongs and a saw all made of iron were also discovered but these along with many more similar objects have been described as trade tools or for domestic utilities.

It is worth mentioning that the earliest surgical instruments that have been discovered are claimed to belong to the Aegean civilisation of about 1400 BCE.[114] These were discovered as a hoard in 1971 and are all made of bronze.

---

[114] Arnott R. 'Surgical practice in the prehistoric Aegean', *Medizinhist J*, 1997; 32: pp. 249-78.

Although their use purely as surgical instruments is a matter of speculation, it is possible that these may be trade implements. But they belong to such a remote antiquity when the tools of trade were usually borrowed for the use in surgery.[115] The maximum number of surgical instruments come from the period of Roman Empire, although from the time of the fall of Roman Empire in about 5th century CE the archaeological discoveries of such objects even from Roman cites appears to be significantly reduced. It would be correct to say that out side Greco-Roman civilisation Gandhara is the only other civilisation where the archaeological excavations have revealed surgical instruments. Since the Greek and Roman surgical artefacts were known to be the only genuine surgical instruments ever discovered; these objects have acquired a place as gold standard for others to be judged or compared with. In this sense the surgical instruments excavated in Gandhara must be weighed against the existing Greek and Roman instruments if these have to be evaluated to establish their authenticity as tools used by the surgeons of Gandhara.

[115] See note 3 above, pp. 21-22.

10.
Surgical instruments excavated in Taxila.

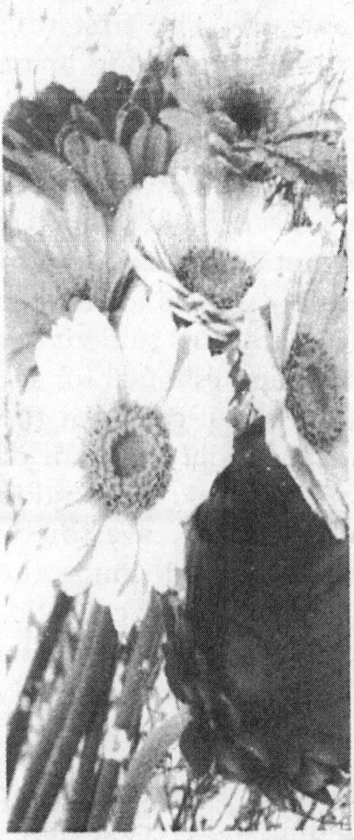

The premise that if an ancient site was associated with substantial historical milieu for the prevalence of organised surgical practise, it increases the likelihood of finding related implements during the archaeological explorations. As for as Gandhara is concerned all the stipulations of such a proposition are fully satisfied. As discussed above with regard to Taxila the history fully supports its association with medicine and surgery. The first related objects were excavated in Taxila during a long phase of archaeological excavations from 1913 to about 1945. This activity was supervised by Sir John Marshall, who after leaving Cambridge became Director General of Archaeological Survey of India. The three volumes that he published on the subject detailing the history and meticulous cataloguing of all what was discovered are worthy witness for his pioneering work and academic high standard. Any student of Gandhara will find his writings valuable and essential for sound understanding of the subject. The significance of the artefacts that he discovered when put under the light of his vast historical knowledge revealed a whole new outlook. After Taxila he went on to supervise excavations at Harappa and Mohenjodaro and published similar three volumes which are also considered most reliable collection of the wholesome facts of archaeology of this amazing civilisation that flourished during 2500 to 2000 BCE.

Sir John Marshall laid the foundation stone of the Taxila museum in 1918, which is surrounded by a pleasant garden (Fig.14). The building was erected close to the major three cities that were excavated, to accommodate the finds at a convenient easily accessible place for the public as well as the archaeologists. The museum building can be reached by the train and road. The museum entrance is appropriately decorated with a picture of Sir John Marshall that every visitor can see on the right side in the entrance hall. From here you enter in to the main hall, there are further two halls for exhibits on either sides of the main hall. In all over 7000 objects are exhibited, which may be categorized into sculptures, coins, jewellery, domestic and trade items. Pottery is also seen in huge numbers along with tools and implements, weapons and many more miscellaneous artefacts. The surgical instruments can be seen in a special glass cabinet in the hall situated on the right side from the main hall. This small museum, rich in the quality of its exhibits is the only place in the World where the only surgical instruments discovered out side the Greek and Roman lands may be seen.

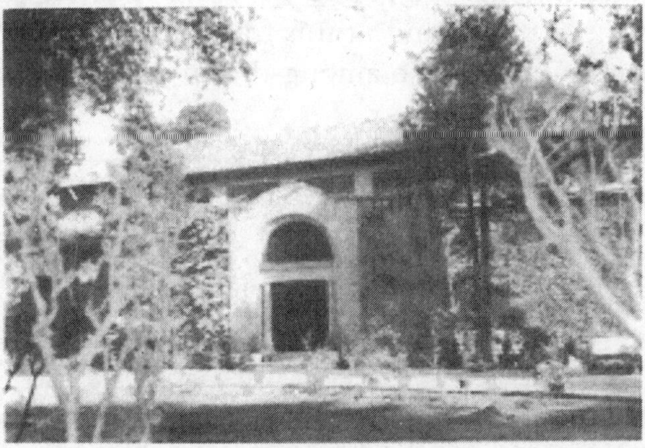

Fig.14
The Taxila museum built in 1918.

One additional feature of the museum is that it is surrounded by a well maintained pleasant garden where many matured trees, shrubs and colourful flowers may be seen. A little away from the museum building stands an old colonial rest house, which must have used by Sir John Marshall and many other famous archaeologists who were involved in the excavations between the wars.

The museum at present displays thirteen objects in the hall, all are exhibited in one place. One object included among these exhibits under the label of surgical instruments is only a handle fragmented from an unknown object or it may be broken off from a surgical instrument because the shape and design of this fragment that is about 10.5 cm in length fits in the shape and design of other instruments (Fig. 15). Although it is also made of pure copper similar to the other surgical instruments, still it cannot be described with certainty as a fragment from a real surgical instrument. It is possible that it may be a broken off piece from either a trade item or from a domestic utensil because many such items made of copper are among the exhibits. The chief difference between this fragment handle and the handles of other surgical instruments is that on cross section it is square shaped while all other handles belonging to the surgical instruments are round on cross section. A typical Buddhist motif at the end of this fragment may also be the reason why it was include among the surgical instruments.

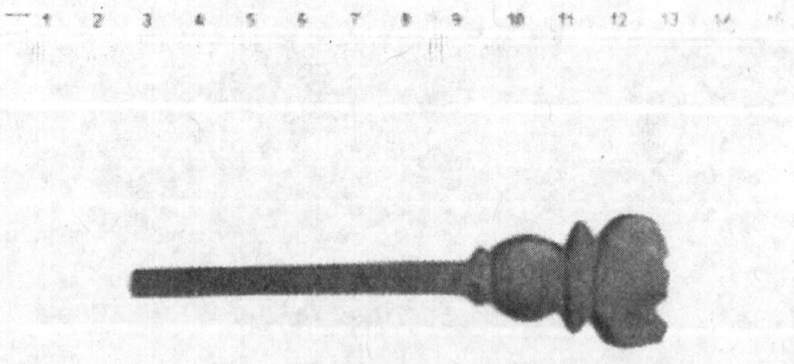

Fig.15

A fragment from an unknown object included among the surgical instrument

Among the remaining objects from the exhibits of Taxila museum that are labelled and displayed under surgical instruments is yet one more object, which in fact is not a surgical instrument and incorrectly placed among the surgical instruments (Fig.16). This is a religious implement that was used by the elder Monk of a monastery or master of ceremonies to present the offerings or donations to gods during sacred rituals.[116] Perhaps it has been included among the surgical instruments for it similarity to the other spatulas.

Fig. 16
This ritual implement has been wrongly included among the surgical instruments

The catalogue does not list all surgical instruments or medical implements in one place but follow its own system of describing and documentation of the discoveries. In order to locate surgical items or other similar objects one has to search the catalogue in a systemic fashion by first searching the illustrations from volume II, then find the description, the site of its discovery in relation to depth in the soil giving an indication of their period from the volume III. At least two surgical instruments included in the display are not in the catalogue and were obviously discovered during the later excavations. Since there are no published catalogues of objects discovered from the time of excavations carried out after John Marshall's departure from Taxila, any archaeological details of these instruments is not available. This also leads to the plausible speculation that some more items must have been discovered but due to lack of strict discipline of cataloguing or absence of an archaeologist with medical interest were not preserved and probably lost. It must be emphasised that this is merely a speculation based on the fact that owing to more awareness few more surgical

---

[116] See note 33 above, vol. 2, p. 595.

instruments have been identified at the newly discovered Buddhist site only a few miles north of Taxila.

The twelve items including the one described above, which is a religious or a ritual device are all grouped together and are illustrated here (Fig.17). The fact that all these historically interesting objects are made of almost pure copper was established by chemical analysis soon after they were discovered. They also retain a distinct patina which makes them appear darkish when seen in artificial light inside the museum; this feature gives them a look of bronze similar to the Roman instruments in the artificial light of the museums. But when taken into natural light they acquire different sheen that of copper, this contrast was clearly noticeable to the author and in the picture of the group of instruments in figure 17 below photographed in natural light such a feature is also visible.

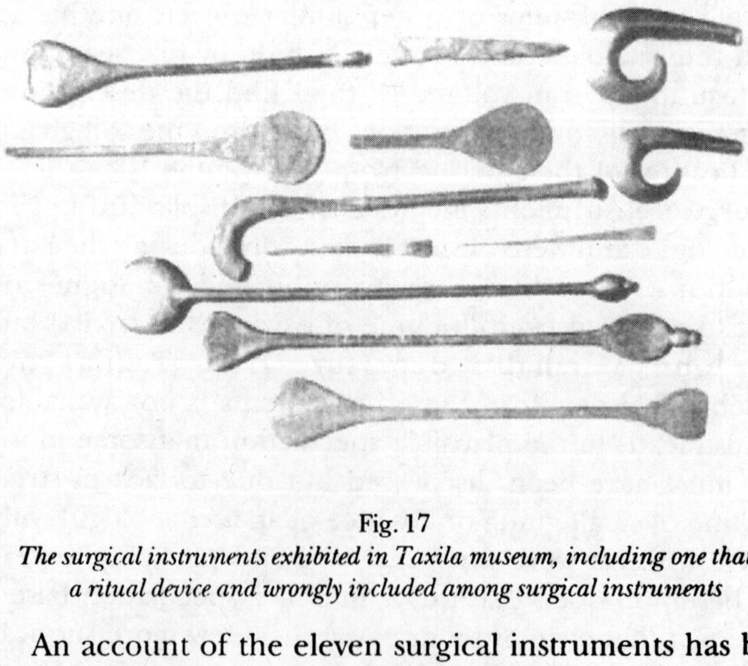

Fig. 17

The surgical instruments exhibited in Taxila museum, including one that is a ritual device and wrongly included among surgical instruments

An account of the eleven surgical instruments has been previously published by the author establishing their merits in a short paper published in 2003.[117] In the forthcoming pages these are now subjected to an enhanced and comprehensive appraisal by more thorough comparison with the Greek and Roman instruments. Nonetheless it must be emphasised that these eleven items are not the only instruments that were discovered in the early excavations of Taxila. A careful search of the catalogue reveals there were some more medical items that appear in the illustrations but are not among the exhibits. The whereabouts of such items listed and illustrated in the catalogue is not known, some may be hidden in the depository access to which was not possible. If they have been lost then it would be most unfortunate tragedy simply because they cannot be replaced. The only consolation is that few of these have been preserved in the illustrations that may be seen in the catalogue. In the following pages an account of each of these eleven surgical instruments follows and all are individually compared with a known Greek or Roman instrument.

Decapitators

The most interesting instruments discovered in Taxila excavations were a number of devices which were identified as decapitators by some experts to whom John Marshall approached for guidance. In view of their significance it is desirable to examine these instruments in greater details. A decapitator is a relatively modern term applied to an obstetric instrument used in the hopeless situation when the foetus has already died in the womb and its head has passed the birth canal but the delivery of rest of the body due to various pertinent reasons cannot be achieved. In ancient times such a clinical problem was not an uncommon complication during the last stages of the birth of a child. The frequency of such incident must be high because an instrument to deal with this difficult situation has been used by many ancient surgeons. Such an instrument has been described in some

[117] Naqvi NH. 'Surgical instruments in the Taxila museum', *Medical History*, 2003; 47: pp. 89-98.

details by many from ancient times to the 10th century CE and remained in use till middle of the 20th century. The archaic writers have also discussed not only similar management but also comparable instruments to deal with this desperate urgency during childbirth. Their recommendation to severe the head using a special instrument and then facilitate the delivery of the remaining dead foetus remained a standard practice for over two thousands years. The fitting name of decapitator was first used by the British obstetrician Ramsbottom during the middle of the nineteenth century.[118] His instrument called Ramsbottom's decapitating hook and another modification with the name of Jardine's decapitating hook remained in use till middle of the twentieth century and may be seen in the surgical instrument catalogues published during 1960s. A further British modification introduced later was Ramsbottom decapitating hook with serrated or saw-toothed in place of sharp inner edge. The Europeans on the other hand described similar devices used for the same purpose but retaining the ancient Roman name of 'hook knife' or 'embryo hook'. The Germans gave it a name of 'Scharfer Haken' or sharp hook.[119] The use of these instruments was discontinued only during later half of the twentieth century when modern methods were introduced in the management of childbirth that eliminated such complication mostly by performing caesarean section more often, vigilant monitoring and other preventive methods.

There is enough convincing evidence that shows that in the remote past the decapitators or sharp hook knives were recommended by various authorities and used during the circumstances described above. The earliest unambiguous reference may be found in *Susruta Samhita*, where a large

---

[118] Hibbard B. *The obstetrician's armamentarium*, San Antonio CA: Norman Publishing, 2000, pp. 254-55.

[119] Kuhn W, Trihler U. eds., *Armamentarium obstetricium Gottingense*, Gottingen: Vandenhoeck and Ruprecht, 1987, p. 119.

part of a chapter is devoted to the surgical management for the removal of dead foetus and other similar calamitous complications during childbirth.[120] It is obvious from the following quote that the urgency to employ such drastic measure was dictated by the primary concern to save the life of the mother while the foetus has already perished is obvious from the following quote from *Susruta Samhita.*

> An intelligent physician should not waste a moment in drawing out the foetus, as soon as it found to be dead in the womb, since neglect in such cases leads to the instantaneous death of the mother, like an animal dying of suffocation. An erudite physician, well versed in anatomy, should use in such cases a *mandalagra* instrument for the purpose of cutting out (the foetus), since a sharp-edged vrddhi-patra may some times hurt the mother during the operation.

The core essence contained in this paragraph from wise Susruta is absolutely clear and cannot be interpreted in any other way. But the statement has introduced one more instrument; this must be investigated to find out exactly what this was and why one has been recommended and the other discouraged. The *mandaḷagra* has been described as an instrument similar to decapitator or a curved knife by another author after discussing various instruments that can be used in obstetrics.[121] While a vrddhi-patra is a straight sharp knife, which obviously would be an absolutely unsuitable and dangerous instrument for use in the circumstances described above.

In the chapter *Sarirasthana* of *Caraka Samhita* operative treatment to remove the dead foetus has been advised in a very brief and passing allusion without giving the details or name of any instrument.

When we look into the *Astangasangraha* of Vagbhata we find much greater details when this destructive procedure

---

[120] Bhishagranta KK. ed. and tr., *Susruta Samhita* (3 volumes), Varanasi: Chowkhamba Sanskrit Series Office, 1981, vol 2, p. 407.

[121] See note 105 above, pp. 1-4.

has to be carried out, detailing the strict indications, instruments to be used and means of hygiene adopted after the operation.[122] The description in *Astangasangraha* is a little more in details than in *Susruta Samhita* as authenticated by the quote below.

> The woman should be consoled, the head of the foetus should be cut either with mandalagra sastra or a anguli sastra (finger knife), the foetus pulled out by holding at its chin, palate, chest or axilla with a grabha sanku (foetal hook); if the head is not cut it should be pulled out by holding at its eye sockets. If impacted by its shoulder (it should be pulled out after) cutting of the arms, if impacted with bloated abdomen resembling an inflated bag, the abdomen should be incised, the intestines pulled out making the abdomen flat and then the foetus pulled out; if impacted by the pelvis, the pelvic bones should be cut and foetus pulled out... Next the *apapa* (placenta) should be brought out by adopting the methods described earlier. In this way the impacted foreign body should be removed and the genitals washed with warm water.

The foremost Roman surgeon Aulus Cornelius Celsus (early to mid first century CE) flourished about the same period when Gandhara and its capital Taxila was at the peak of its advancement and important visitors from Roman Empire were known to have travelled to Taxila. In his well known book *De Medicina* Celsus has also elaborated the complexities of the difficult clinical situation when as a result of obstructed labour the foetus has died inside the womb. The name Celsus has used for a special instrument in such situation is *Uncus qui* or a sharp hook for cutting the head of a dead foetus by severing at the neck. After a thorough discussion with emphasis on the seriousness of the situation signifying the urgency and deep concern for saving the life of the mother he recommended surgical treatment in the following words.[123]

---

[122] See note 94 above, vol ii, p. 54.

[123] Spenser WG. ed. and tr., *Celsus De Medicina*, London: William Heinemann, 1938, pp. 459-60.

> The remedy then is to cut the neck, in order that the two parts may be extracted separately. This is done with a hook which resembles the one mentioned above, but has all its inner edge sharp. Then we must proceed to extract the head first and then the rest.

Soranus of Ephesus (98-138 CE) was the first to write a comprehensive text on obstetrics in which the procedure of embryotomy or surgical removal of the foetus that has died before birth has been described in some details. It is recommended to use a specially made embryo hooks, though Soranus in his text has not made any distinction between blunt or sharp hooks.[124] The teachings of Soranus were followed by Aetius of Amida in the sixth century CE and lastly Paul of Agineta during the seventh century CE; both of them advise embryotomy in similar clinical circumstances.[125] But none of these two authors mention name of any specific instruments that can be used in the operations they recommend.

After Roman and Byzantium medical writers the first Arab who contributed a major work in surgery was Albucasis (died 1013) who wrote a massive text *At-Tasrif,* which contains most comprehensive details on surgery.[126] It must be the first book of its kind where illustrations of many surgical instruments appear as the author himself has described these devices, a fact we can ourselves judge from its earliest Latin translations preserved in many libraries. The all-inclusive details in the chapter dealing with obstetrics and drawings of a number of hooks and sharp curved knives seen in the available manuscripts; leaves us in no doubt that sharp hook knives were part of Albucasis armamentarium. One

[124] Temkin O. tr., *Soranus's Gynecology,* Baltimore: Johns Hopkins University Press, 1956, pp. 189-97.

[125] Adams F. tr., *The seven books of Paulus Aegineta* (3 volumes), London: Sydenham Society, 1844-1847, vol. I, p. 648.

[126] Spink MS, Lewis GL. trs, *Albucassis surgery and instruments,* London: Wellcome Institute of the History of Medicine, 1973.

such hook has been included in figure 21, where all known decapitators seen in collections or appear in texts are collected together for comparison with each other.[127] The vital information that cannot be derived from the illustrations of the surgical instruments in various manuscripts of Albucasis is about the size of the instruments. Although, Spink who has translated Albucasis from original Arabic into English in 1971, in an earlier paper suspected whether the sharp hook was known to Albucasis?[128] It is also desirable to emphasise here that no surgical instruments of Arab origin comparable to the drawings seen in about 50 known manuscripts of Albucasis have ever been discovered in archaeological excavations. Although for this lack of archaeological evidence there are numerous valid reasons, on the other hand the textual evidence is robust and convincing.

It is worthwhile to examine the decapitators that have been excavated and are displayed in the Taxila museum. The decapitators excavated in Taxila, are the most interesting and unique objects exhibited in Taxila museum. Sir John Marshall who was responsible for the excavations must have taken into consideration opinions of the medical archaeologists before making the following assessment at the time of their discovery.[129]

> The purpose of these curious looking instruments is by no means certain, but the accepted view, which the writer does not share, is that they were surgical decapitators for use in obstetric operations.

In all six such instruments were excavated that are listed and illustrated in the catalogue, but only three may be seen

---

[127] Hamerneh S. 'Drawings and pharmacy in Al-Zahrawi's 10th century surgical treatise', *United States National Museum Bulletin,* Washington DC: Smithsonian Institution, 1961; 228: pp. 81-94.

[128] Spink MS. 'Arabian gynaecological, obstetrical and genito-urinary practice illustrated from Albucasi,' *Proceedings of the Royal society of medicine,* vol. xxx; 1937: pp. 654-71.

[129] See note 33 above, vol 2, pp. 599-601.

exhibited. The other three are probably lost or might be misplaced because two of them were discovered only as fragments approximately 5.5 cm long. They were made from sheets of copper strengthened on outer border with a copper-wire rib. Both fragments were discovered from the earliest site described above as Bhir Mound at the depth that was dated to second century BCE. From this we can derive that such a device was in use in Taxila before the invasion of Alexander. The third decapitator among the three that are now presumably are lost was excavated complete from the site of Sirkap in the layers belonging to first century CE. It was 17.5 cm long, made of solid copper with a round handle and a disc at its end. The pictures of this complete decapitator and one of the fragments described above can be seen in the catalogue but there is no picture of the third fragment.

Among the other three, which are displayed two are only fragments of blades without the handles, although the catalogue shows them with handles that must have been lost at some stage. Their length with the handles had been recorded as 16.5 cm; without the handles they measure about 6 and 7.5 cm (Fig.18). These were discovered at two different sites in Sirkap in layers from first or second century CE. Both appear to be distorted in their shapes possibly due to ageing or metal stress. One seen on the left side of the figure clearly shows a stress related crack in line of stress at its outer border.

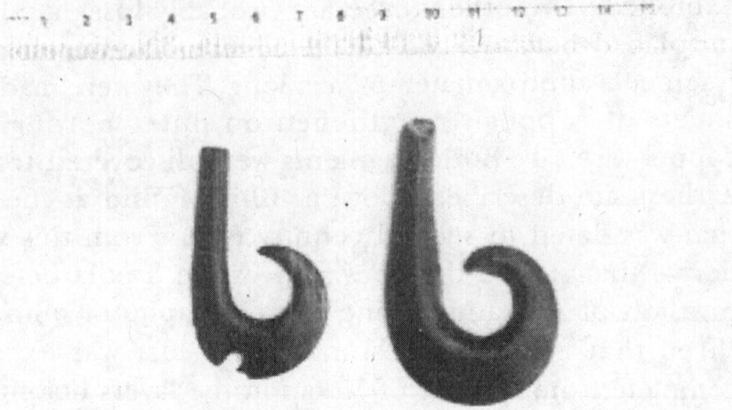

Fig. 18
Two decapitators without handles excavated in Taxila

The third decapitator that can be seen displayed is almost complete except at the terminal end of the blade, which shows some damage and minor loss at the very end and also a crack in metal (Fig.19 and 20). It is a robustly constructed instrument of solid copper. It was discovered in the second stratum in Sirkap that makes it to belong to the first century CE, a period associated with the reign of Kanishka. This very distinctive instrument is 16.5 cm long, having a strong handle which is round on cross section and terminates into a disc at the end. The blade is curved with sharp inner edge and blunt on outer. The handles of all these decapitators discovered in Taxila resemble the handle of this particular instrument. All have few unique features that are common to all of them irrespective of their period. They are made of solid copper, in length they are uniformly 16.5-17 cm long, the handles are round in cross section and terminate into a disc. When held in hand this ancient excavated device gives a feel of a balanced workable instrument.

Fig. 19
An almost complete decapitator from Taxila

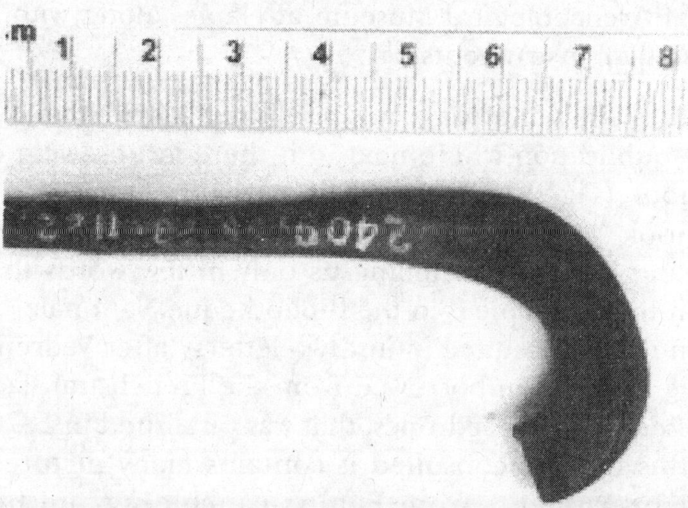

Fig. 20
A close up of the above decapitator

A comparative account of embryo hooks that have been excavated from Roman and Byzantine sites would be a useful exercise in evaluating the decapitators described above that have been excavated in Taxila. Benedetto Vulpes during first half of the nineteenth century was probably the first medical archaeologist who studied the surgical instruments discovered from various sites of Pompeii. About these discoveries he made a number of communications to the Royal Academy of Archaeology during 1846. In 1847 he published his book in an atlas style which portrayed the excavated surgical instruments including a Roman embryo hook in its real size.[130] The description of this instrument matched perfectly with the embryo hook described by Celsus in *De Medicina*. Although Vulpes did not make any differentiation between sharp or blunt embryo hooks. The Pompeii embryo hook was described by Vulpes to be 17 cm long, and its handle was made of copper alloy, the sharp hook was of iron. Its present length is only 7.7 cm because the iron hook has been rusted away while the handle made of bronze remains intact. This object is now exhibited at the National Archaeological Museum at Naples along with five other similar instruments.[131]

In 1907 the same image was published by J S Milne in his famous publication where next to it there is a drawing of a sharp hook (Fig. 21).[132] About this particular drawing of the sharp hook Milne has recorded rather ambiguous or even misleading information telling us only in few words that a knife on this principle is in the Bibliotheque Nationale. The diagram itself is credited in just two letters, 'after Vèdrènes', implying it has been borrowed from the French translation of *De Medicina* by A. Vèdrènes, that was published in 1876.[133] But if this book is consulted it contains many pictures of Roman instruments from Pompeii including the hook described by Vulpes but no diagram of a sharp hook similar

---

[130] Vulpes B. *Illustrazione di Tutti gli strumenti chirurgici Scavati in Erolano e in Pompei*, Napoli: Stamperia Reale, 1847, p. 81.

[131] Bliquez LJ. *Roman surgical instruments and other minor objects in the National Archaeological Museum of Naples*, Mainz: Verlag Philipp von Zabern, 1994, pp. 129-30.

[132] Milne JS. *Surgical instruments in Greek and Roman times*, Oxford: Clarendon Press, 1907, p. 154.

[133] Vèdrènes A. tr., *Traité de médicine de AC Celse*, Paris: G Masson, 1876.

to one depicted by Milne can be seen in the referred publication. It seems that the drawing was Milne's own, made from the description he found in the French translation of *De Medicina.* Nevertheless the drawing turns into an important testimony since it is the only representation of a Roman sharp hook because no Roman sharp hook as described by Celsus and illustrated by Milne has ever been excavated.

During the search of various catalogues a sharp embryo hook of Byzantine origin was located in the publication of German scholar Ernst Künzl, who has illustrated a hook labelled as *Großer Haken* (great hook).[134] This object is in the collection at Schiller University in Jena in Germany. It was excavated from a well known Byzantine site in Turkey and appears remarkably similar to the decapitator from Taxila.

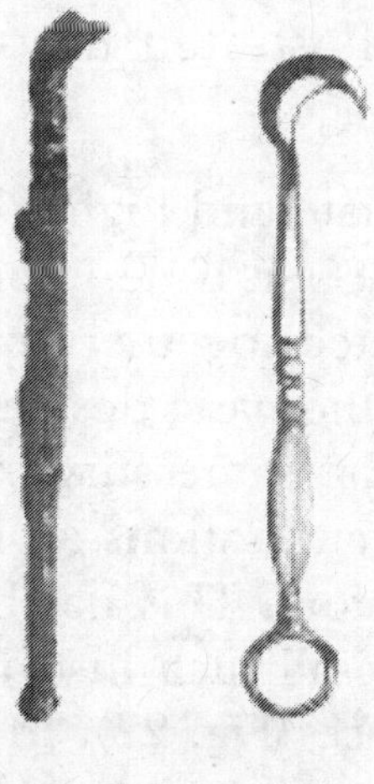

Fig. 21
Embryo hook from Pompeii and drawing of a Roman sharp hook (as depicted by Milne)

From the analysis of the references and quotes that have been cited in the above discussion it is abundantly clear that in a frantic situation when the foetus has already been lost or died inside the womb, the life of the mother is in grave

[134] Künzl E. *Medizinische Instrumente aus Sepulkralfunden der römischen Kaiserzeit,* Cologne: Rheinland, 1983, p. 52.

danger a piecemeal removal or embryotomy of the foetus was fully justified. The procedure was carried out during the ancient times by severing the neck of the foetus and in order to minimise injury to the mother, Roman surgeons used a hook like instrument that was sharp on the inside border and blunt out side. It was modified from the Roman blunt hook, which they already had in their armamentarium that was used to extract the limb of foetus during difficult child birth. They called the modified instrument a sharp hook. It had a strong handle made of bronze attached to a blade made of iron that was sharp inside and blunt out side. Their description recorded in ancient texts and discovery of similar instruments in archaeological finds confirms its use throughout the ancient obstetric practice. The decapitators discovered in Taxila are comparable with the sharp embryo hook that has been described from Celsus to Albucasis and even illustrated in various catalogues of instruments of recent age.

In order to appreciate and highlight the close similarity of these historical devices it is desirable that all the known devices may be illustrated together and a visual assessment is made to figure out the basic design of such devices that have been used for the same surgical procedure by the surgeons of different civilisations all through the last two thousands years of history. This has been achieved in the next illustration, where all such instruments are assembled side by side in one place (Fig. 22). In this picture only the modern decapitators on the right side of the picture are shown with a scale, others are not to scale but the lengths of these are known except for one that has been adopted from Albucasis. The lengths of others have been recorded along with their description in the main text. It should also be pointed out that the various modern catalogues list at least seven other decapitators of British, American and European design but they are so modern that a comparison with ancient instruments will not be justified and these are not included in present discussion. The two decapitators from mid nineteenth century illustrated at right hand side of the figure make a fair comparison with ancient ones.

Finally it is crucial to record that although a Roman sharp hook has never been discovered in excavations, it is probable that among the five hooks without blades displayed in the National Archaeological Museum at Naples one might belong to a sharp hook.

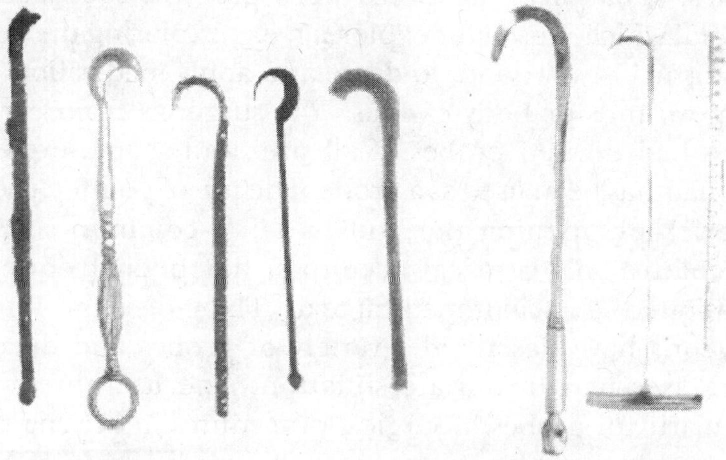

A B C D E F G

Fig 22

A. Roman embryo hook excavated in Pompeii, first described by Vulpes.
B. Sharp hook illustrated by JS Milne in his publication.
C. Byzantine embryo hook in the Jena collection, Germany.
D. Hook knife from a manuscript of Albucasis
E. Decapitator excavated in Taxila.
F. Ramsbottom's decapitator.
G. Jardine's decapitator.

Probes

A probe may be considered as an extension of the finger used as a multipurpose device in every day setting. Probes made of stone, wood, horns, bone, ivory and all sort of metals have been discovered in archaeological excavations among all civilisations. They were discovered in make-up boxes of the Egyptian ladies and can also be seen in Gandhara sculptures where a lady is depicted in a posture of enhancing the attraction of her eyes by applying kohl using a probe like device, a popular practice very well alive and prevalent even today. Probes and hair pins for fashion statement have been discovered in large numbers in Taxila.

In medical setting the probe is a basic or primary form of an instrument that has been used from earliest times to this day to feel, explore, diagnose and treat in multitudes of clinical situations. The Greek word probe is equivalent of 'sound' which is used for exploring, e.g. exploring the depth of a fistula or a wound, to dilate and apply medication into deep wounds or body cavities. The surgeons from earliest times had devised probes of all sizes and shape, even the hog hair has been used as a probe. The use of pointed probes to prick or opening the boils, a fairly common surgical procedure in historical accounts, has been frequently mentioned in ancient medical texts. The Greek and Roman surgeons have described a variety of probes and detailed their uses in appropriate situation. The usefulness and popularity of probes in surgical procedures indicating their extensive use is also represented in the discovery of large number of these instruments from Greek and Roman sites, now seen in museums or catalogues.

Probes are also described in *Susruta Samhita* by its Sanskrit name *Salaka* meaning a rod, a name representative of the shape not the function as we have noticed in its Greek equivalent. In Susruta Samhita the probe has been described in following words.[135]

> The *Salaka* (rod) should be made of to measure eight fingers in length, its middle part being covered with strings of thread and resembling the upper section of the thumb in circumference and its ends terminating in the form of a bud. The *Salaka* should be prepared from copper, iron or gold.

[135] See note 120 above, vol III, p. 81.

There are three copper probes in the Taxila collection, which have not been rerecorded by Marshall in his catalogue of excavations indicating that these must have been discovered at a later date. The two have pointed ends on one side and flattened on other, these are approximately 7 cm and 9 cm long both are delicately made of pure copper (Fig. 23). These were most probably utilised for puncturing or lancing a boil, explorations of a wound or fistula and the flat ends were for application of medication in deeper places. The third probe may be seen in the group where all the instruments are illustrated above. It is a 6.5 cm long blunt instrument; the correct shape of its ends cannot be ascertained due to marked wear and tear. Susruta has mentioned a probe shaped like an earthworm; this description might fit to this object if it was not badly damaged and also to the rounded end of smaller probe in figure 22. All these three probes are comparable to various Roman probes that have been illustrated in different catalogues and seen in Museums. Some of the Roman probes have olivary end on one side, which is similar to a bud shaped probe described in *Susruta Samhita,* though no probe of this shape and description is in Taxila collection. Nevertheless there are numerous styli or metal pens used for writing purposes, kohl rods and pins that can also be used as probes. As for as metal styli or pens are concerned Milne tells us that they being at hand and suitable shaped were often used as surgical instruments. The two probes described above when compared with a Roman probe are unmistakably similar (Fig. 24); this instrument has been illustrated by Milne in his book.[136]

[136] See note 132 above, plate III, figure 1a.

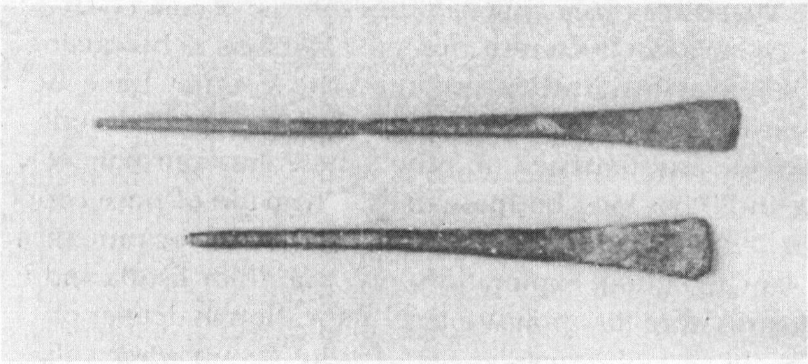

Fig. 23
Two copper probes from Taxila

Fig. 24
A 7.5 cm long Roman Probe (Milne)

Spatulae

Spatulae have been used for surgical, pharmaceutical and also for a variety of non medical purposes in the remote past. The spatulae excavated from Greek and Roman sites were quite substantial and make the largest representation in numbers. Many of these were made to perform dual function where one end was made into an olivary probe and the other as spatula. It is also mentioned that originally they were used to scoop and apply medication such as ointments or other similar substances to the body and gradually were adopted for other medical uses and even in surgical procedures as retractors.

In the catalogue of the Taxila excavations there are five spatulae listed among the surgical instruments, all bear an unmistakable decoration or motif of Buddhist *nandipada* that in fact renders the free end worthless for any another useful purpose, a significant difference when compared with the

Roman design of dual purpose spatulae. One spatula in the above mentioned catalogue is unique having a heart shaped hole in its blade the purpose of which is unclear, it may simply be decorative. Three out of five of the spatulae that were discovered are missing while the remaining two are displayed in the museum (Fig. 25 and 26). Both have an oval shaped flattened blade end and decoration on the free end of the handle, they are about 20 to 22 cm in length and are made of solid copper, no damage can be noticed anywhere, they are robust and not malleable. All the five spatulae were discovered from Sirkap in depths associated with the first or second century CE. It is not possible to find an instrument described in the Sanskrit medical texts that might resemble a spatula but translators of few of these texts have described a spoon shaped instrument without giving information about its size or other attributes that might give us any speculative hints to connect it with the spatulae discovered in Taxila. These two objects not just in physical appearance but functionally as well resemble many of the Roman spatulae we see in various catalogues. As an example the two illustrated in figures 25 and 26 may be compared with many shown in figures 107-144 illustrated by Bliquez in his catalogue of Roman surgical instruments in the National Archaeological Museum of Naples.[137] One 18 cm long similar instrument with olivary end from Milne's publication is illustrated below (fig. 27) for the sake of comparison with the two spatulae from Taxila.[138]

---

[137] Bliquez LJ. *Roman surgical instruments and other minor objects in the National Archaeological Museum of Naples,* Mainz: Verlag Philipp Von Zabern, 1994, pp. 135-44.

[138] See note 132 above, plate XIII, figure 1.

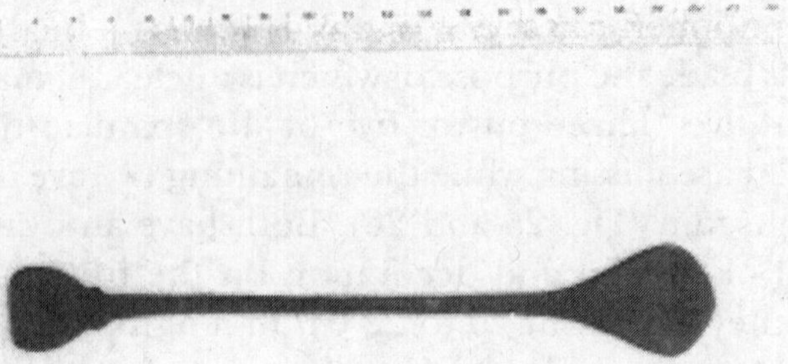

Fig. 25
A spatula displayed in the Taxila

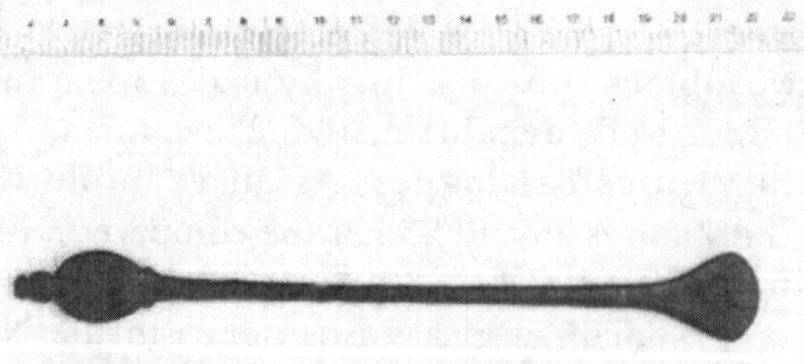

Fig. 26
The second spatula in Taxila museum

Fig. 27
18 cm long Roman spatula (Milne)

Tongue Depressors

The remaining three instruments illustrated in the group of instruments above are not listed nor do their pictures appear any where in the catalogue. It is presumed they were also discovered during later excavations. All three are similar in shape but two are about 13 cm and 14 cm long while the third has much smaller handle measuring only 9 cm. They have flattened oval blades and rounded handles without any decorations at the end. All three are made of solid copper. These have been described as tongue depressors and also resemble with similar Roman instruments. The smaller one and one of the larger one are illustrated below (Fig. 28 and 29). A Roman tongue depressor is also portrayed after these two which in general shape and size makes fair comparison with the instruments excavated in Taxila (Fig. 30).

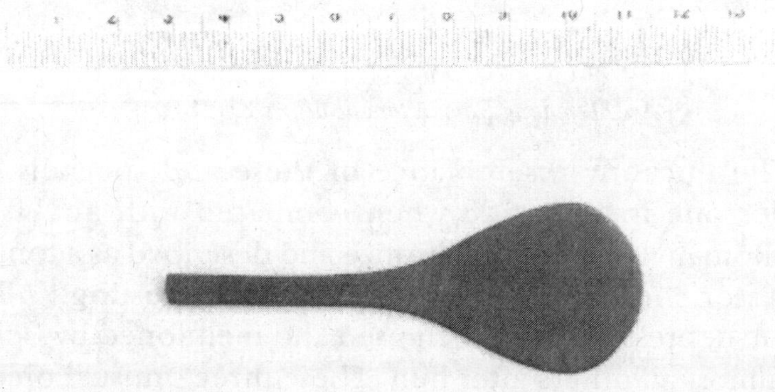

Fig. 28
Small tongue depressor from Taxila 9 cm long

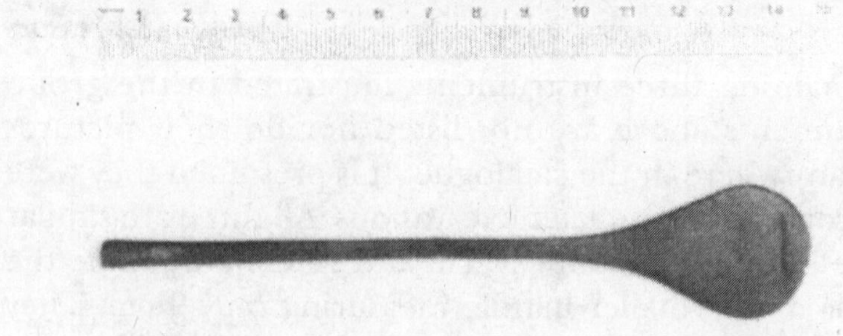

Fig. 29
One of the two larger tongue depressors from Taxila 13 cm long

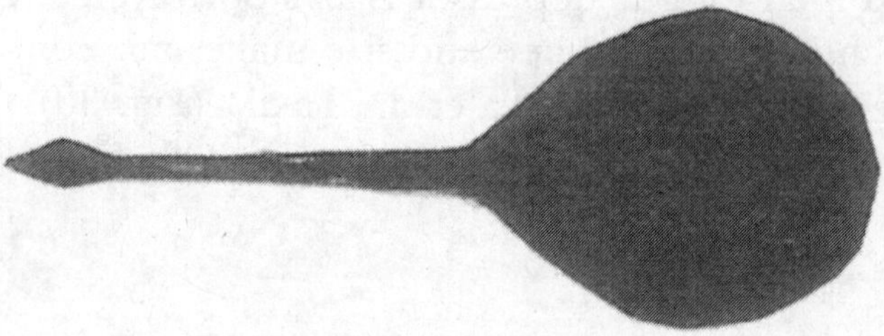

Fig. 30
An 11cm long Roman tongue depressor (Milne)

The uncanny resemblance of these and specially the smaller one in figure 28 when compared with an 11 cm long Roman instrument of bronze and described as a tongue depressor shown above in figure 30 is interesting.[139] The tongue depressors have been used and mentioned by Celsus and almost all others after him. These three unusual objects from Taxila in shape, design and weight are completely different from many other domestic and trade appliances in the collection. The location of their find and the exact period or layers they were excavated from is not known. Their use as tongue depressors is highly plausible because such instruments have also been described in the major Sanskrit medical texts and their semblance with known Roman tongue depressors when compared with the known

[139] See note 132 above, plate XX, figure 6.

Roman tongue depressors as illustrated above is unmistakable.

This completes the account of those objects which were excavated at different times and may be seen today displayed together as surgical instruments in one display cabinet in the eastern hall of the Taxila museum. Their significance being the only surgical instruments discovered in archaeological excavations other than the Greek and Roman sites is significant for the students of history of Buddhism and history of medicine in India in general. Their local design also gives unequivocal support to the historical evidence for surgical practice in Buddhist Gandhara that was at par with the Roman surgical practice during the immediate pre and post centuries of the Christian era.

Now we may look into those instruments and medical artefacts that were excavated and they have been described in apt details in the extensive catalogues prepared by Sir John Marshall but are not seen displayed any where in the Taxila museum. It is not possible to report that some of these may be hidden in the depository because the author was not able to access the depository despite repeated requests. The other worrying likelihood that the absent objects have been lost or stolen over the long period from the time of their discovery is also not certain but remains a probability. The illegal antique market where Gandhara art is bought and sold is a flourishing business in all the western countries. The uncouth dealers take full advantage of the poverty and weaknesses in the host countries and of prolonged political upheaval when controls are impossible. Such a state of affairs gives them godsend opportunities to exploit the situation paying peanuts to those who can steal to order even from the museum displays. Apart from important large sculptures minor metal objects from Gandhara like coins, pins, rods for kohl application are often seen in antique shops, auction houses or even advertised on the internet. It is difficult to distinguish if any surgical instruments are included among those offered by the sellers who invariably deal in illegally acquired objects. There is almost no organised monitoring against the day light robberies. The situation has gone out of proportion during the last 20 years due to the disastrous war raging in Afghanistan. The objects that were buried deep under the earth remained protected for thousands of years but sooner they were excavated they have been lost for ever.

Forceps

It has been mentioned elsewhere that tweezers or a pair of forceps was one of the earliest metal instruments ever discovered in archaeological excavations. One was found in about 5000 years old ruins of Ur. A bronze forceps was also among the hoard of tools belonging to the Aegean civilisation. It has also been suggested by various archaeologists and historians that tweezers or surgical forceps were interchangeable in ancient times and the same instrument was used for both purposes when needed. A number of specially constructed forceps have been excavated from different Roman sites which were used to adjust the wicks of the oil lamps. These are displayed in the British Museum. These discoveries offer sufficient verification that a pair of forceps was one of the earliest implements invented by humans that was used not only as surgical instrument but also utilised in many other domestic and trade pursuits.

When searching for a forceps from the Taxila excavations we are not disappointed. One pair of forceps that was discovered here demands careful attention. It was made from a long single copper band, bent in the middle and then strengthened with another piece of copper ring near to the loop (Fig. 31). This design also provided some strength and extra springiness to the instrument. This pair of forceps is 8 cm long and was found in stratum II belonging to early first century BCE. It was discovered in the Greek township of Sirkap of Taxila. This particular object was described by Sir John Marshall himself as surgical forceps while others similar objects made of iron were listed as tweezers elsewhere in the catalogue. The pair of forceps discovered from Taxila is again similar to many such instruments of Greek and Roman origin that may be seen in most European museums or catalogues. In order to make comparison with a similar object, which is also 8 cm long and comes from a well known Greek site, both are illustrated side by side in figure 31. The forceps of Greek origin is exhibited in the museum of Epidaurus and its use as surgical instrument is in no doubt because it was discovered among many other bronze instruments in the grave of a doctor. Moreover Epidaurus is famous site where god of healing was supposed to reside and it was a centre where people came to seek treatment for their ailments.

The surgical forceps have been described by both Susruta and Vagbhata in their massive manuscripts and there is strong indication that such objects were also used for epilating purposes.[140] Although there seems to be no sculptural depiction of forceps being used in the act of make up in thc Gandhara art.

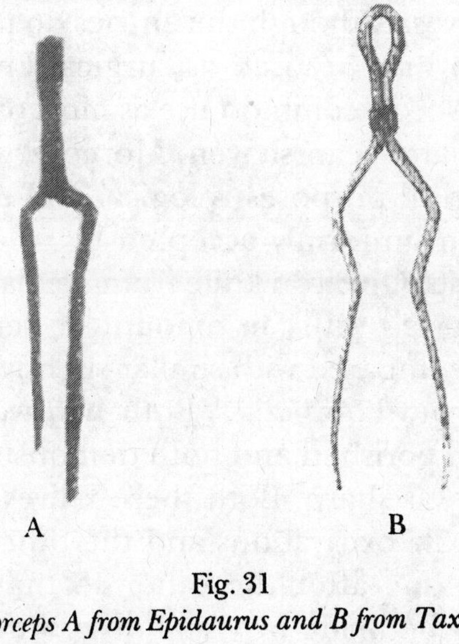

A B

Fig. 31

Forceps A from Epidaurus and B from Taxila

[140] See note 107 above, pp. 79-80.

Scalpels

Leaving aside the exact period all the three major medical texts of Caraka, Susruta and Vagbhata have described a variety of surgical knives along with their names and most of the time they are careful to mention the size measured in fingers. In view of the fact that Taxila was a medical centre the presence of surgical knife in Gandhara is not surprising. Why lot more were not discovered must be because the delicate and sharp objects made of iron were rusted out and many knives or similar objects have not survived. Moreover it is not possible to distinguish between a domestic, hunting or surgical knife from those excavated in badly damaged conditions, particularly if they remained buried for more than two millennia under the earth. In contrast majority of Roman surgical artefacts were recovered well preserved because they remained protected under the ash of Vesuvius. Such a premise is justifiably applicable to sharp edged objects.

Apparently only few sharp iron objects excavated in Taxila are seen in the catalogue, some of these have been described as knives. Although the entries do not specify their functions, some may be used as surgical knives or razors. The razors must be in common use as most of the sculptures from Gandhara are clean shaven. Moreover use of razors if needed for surgical purposes is logical and use of razors in surgery has been uniformly accepted by medical historians and archaeologists. One iron knife from Taxila, 8 cm in length that is heavily rusted with fair amount of deterioration can be comfortably compared with similar slightly bigger Roman surgical knife from Pompeii.[141] Both had wooden handles which have been perished and both demonstrate a rounded front edge that was sharp. Both these knives, one from the catalogue of Taxila excavations and the other from Milne's text are placed one after the other so that a convincing comparison may be made by visual observation (Fig. 32). It

[141] See note 132 above, plate VII, figure 4.

is strange that the damage due to rust these have suffered also looks uniform and similar.

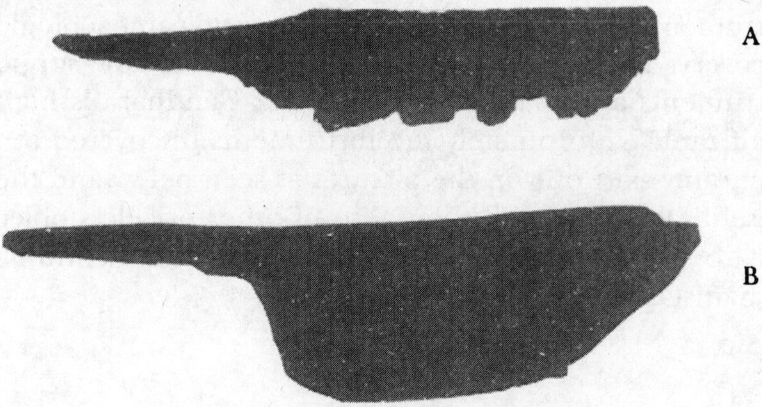

Fig. 32
Heavily rusted and damaged at the sharp edge scalpel or razor from Taxila (A) with a similar Roman (B) blade (Milne)

A few surgical instruments were also discovered in Afghanistan by a French team of archaeologists during 60s and 70s of the last century. This discovery was at the Greek site called Ai Khanoum in the North-Eastern region of Afghanistan.[142] The town was founded by Alexander and probably was named Alexandria. It remained a Greek out post or a colony for many centuries and was destroyed probably by natural catastrophe in about 135 BCE. Among the finds were surgical instruments consisting of two forceps, two spatulae, a suturing needle and a surgical knife, some of these are illustrated here (Fig. 33).[143] All these instruments were made of iron and look like typical Greek or Roman surgical instruments. The knife with longish blade and an olivary handle is particularly significant because it looks exactly the same as many scalpels seen in the museum

[142] Dupree NH. *A historical guide to Afghanistan,* Kabul: Afghanistan Tourist Organization Publication, 1970.

[143] Guillaume O. Rougeulle A. *Fouilles D'Ai Khanoum,* Paris: De Boccard, 1984, Pl. XI, figure 6.

of Naples. These instruments discovered at the site known as the gate through which the Greek took hold of and controlled Gandhara for a long time. The discovery of these instruments at this unique site is an interesting archaeological discovery. The presence of these few unmistakable surgical instruments at a place that was part of Gandhara is highly significant. Unfortunately the instruments discovered at Ai Khanoum exist only in the pictures as seen below and their present fate along with thousands of other priceless objects due to looting during the destruction and turmoil in Afghanistan is not known.

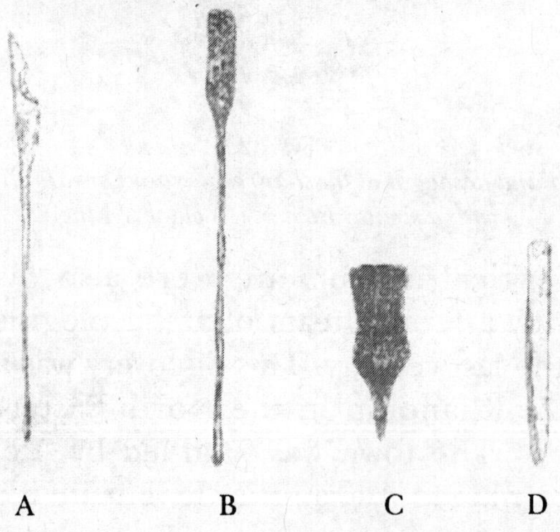

Fig. 33
Surgical instruments excavated at Ai Khanoum in Afghanistan. (From Fouilles D'Ai Khanoum) A= scalpel, B= Spatula. C=fragment of a spatula D=Forceps

Suturing Needles

Needles made from wood, bone, horn and ivory and other substances were known from early Stone Age, due to tiny size and the biodegradable nature many such objects have not survived or discovered during excavations. As technical skill of the people increased needles made of bronze and other than iron have also been discovered in archaeological excavations because these could survive than rust prone iron objects. At what stage of their development the human being started using needles to suture wounds or deep cuts in the skin is difficult to pinpoint but it seems it was a feat achieved at an early period. The needles made of bronze, copper and iron have been excavated though not in great numbers among all civilisations even though they were probably the smallest objects that could survived and discovered buried under the soil for centuries. It is also logical to assume that the needles used for stitching garments made of leather and other material like wool or cotton were also used for suturing wounds when ever required. From the sites of later period of human advance the archaeologists have identified those needles discovered from known graves or houses of surgeons that obviously must have been used for suturing the wounds or to close the incision after surgery. The pertinent features of such needles have not been laid down but those that were found from excavations are usually made of copper, bronze and rarely of iron, having a smaller eye and sometimes the body is triangular on cross section. They appear stronger and sharper than the ordinary needles. A needle made of ivory was found in a surgeon's tool kit; it was for stitching the bandages and was discovered from a Roman site in London.

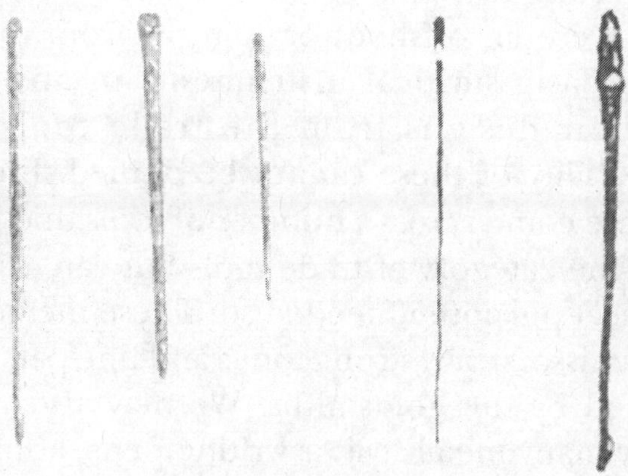

A B C

Fig. 34

Three Suturing needles from Taxila (A) a Roman needle (B) (Milne) and one suturing needle from Ai Khanoum (C)

Although surgical or suturing needles were not identified in the archaeology of pre-Vedic culture such as Mehrgarh (7000 BCE), Harappa and Mohenjodaro but needles for other purposes were in common use. We are further informed by T. A. Wise that needles for the purpose of suturing wounds were used during the time of Rig-Veda.[144] Susruta has given details of repairing the eye lid using fine needle and horse hair as suturing material. This was further elaborated by Vagbhata by advising that the horse hair suture must be removed from the eye lid after five days. The discovery of the three surgical needles from Taxila once more offers support to the data documented in the texts. All these three needles were discovered in the oldest township of Bhir Mound, in layers of second century BCE. The needles from Taxila are placed along with a Roman surgical needle and a Greek needle that was discovered in Ai Khanoum (Fig. 34).

Trade tools that might be used in surgery

In the above discussion it has been mentioned that the ancient surgeons would borrow tools from a carpenter, goldsmith or blacksmith if one that suited his clinical need and not present in his surgical tool box. The surgical instruments were an offshoot or spin off from the tools of trades. The basic surgical instruments in any way have followed their designs from the trade tools and the interchangeability of these cannot be denied. From Taxila excavations we come across a number of tools that have been included in the category of trade tools but can also be used for the surgical purpose if needed so. These include devices like a pair of scissors, saw, strong tongs and fine pair of forceps probably used by the goldsmiths. We may also include in this category many metal styli or writing pens, kohl rods and metal pins or similar other fashion items found in large numbers and readily available in most house hold. Many of

---

[144] See note 104 above, p.171.

these items even as small as the hair pins or dress pins are among the exhibits in Taxila museum, but many more are not exhibited and are only seen in the catalogue. Some other heavier and substantial trade tools were also discovered and their presence further consolidates the notion that in desperate situation they can offer useful aid to a surgeon. Few such objects that could easily be borrowed for surgery are shown in the accompanied picture (Fig. 35). They are all made of iron except the stylus and kohl rod, which are made of copper. This might be the reason or cause of heavy rusting of those objects made of iron and the resulting damage seen as a consequence. Despite damage due to rust the refined design of these objects is also a verification of the skills of manufacturing of the artisans of Gandhara and their competence to design and make tools of trade and surgical instruments for the use of appropriate user.

A B C D E F G

Fig. 35

Some trade objects of iron and copper excavated from Taxila

A. Fragment of a scissor
B. Forceps
C. Tongs
D. Tongs
E. Tongs
F. Stylus
G. Kohl rod

(From Marshall)

11. Pharmaceutical objects

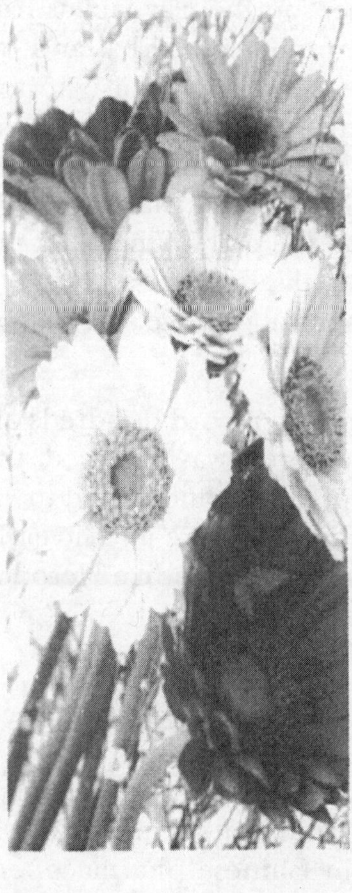

Throughout the ages or from earliest times the therapies that a medicine man could offer were mostly derived from plant or made from herbal ingredients. In due course other materials from animals or inorganic substances were also included in the ever increasing list of medicinal agents. The prescriptions written on the clay tablets from Mesopotamia have recorded a number of herbal and other constituent listed in them, these gives us an insight how important was the art of recognising the plants and combining them together and exploiting them for their healing powers. It would not be wrong to say that during the infancy the medicine walked on the path of the plant pharmacy to reach the maturity. In all civilisations the art of apothecary remained the backbone of medical practice and probably in some what different ways still is.

The Egyptian papyri record hundreds of herbs for which a whole army of gatherers was deployed, then the collected plants were to be prepared and stored in safe containers to be dispensed to those who were ill. The earliest Greek writes like Homer and then historian like Herodotus have praised the superior medical knowledge of Egyptians and their herbal remedies.

In Chinese medicine great deal more constituents from vegetables; mineral and animal origin is used in the therapeutic preparations that are usually taken in much bulky doses than in any other medical system. There are over 5000 plants in Chinese pharmacopoeia that must be stored in a well stocked pharmacy. To this if medicines of mineral and animal origin are included the problem of simple storage becomes a huge challenge, requiring a planed strategy for collection, storage, preparation and eventually dispensing to the end user. The elaborate system of labelling a variety of jars and other ceramic containers has been illustrated in many of the pictures representing a typical Chinese pharmacy. It might be true that the Chinese were so overburdened with their pharmacopoeia that they probably neglected to pay attention to pathology or rational surgery in their system of medicine.

Among the Greeks, Theophrastus (300 BCE) must be considered the first who made a scientific study of plants and specified those plants that had medicinal properties. In the first century CE it was Dioscorides who travelled with the Roman armies far and wide and wrote the earliest text on medical botany in a systemic fashion, his writings were followed by many long after him. After the Greek and Roman decline the Arabs took over, they created organised and grand pharmacies; where the prescriptions were prepared in a standardised and controlled environment, utilising standardised weights and measures. Alberuni tells us that the word used for pharmacy in Arabic language *'Al-saydanah'* is derived from *sandal,* which is taken from Sanskrit word *'chandan'* meaning sandalwood. It entered the vocabulary because in Arabic speaking lands the person selling medicines among other merchandise also had the expensive item sandalwood.[145]

In Ayurvedic system of medicine the prescriptions were prepared with great care by combining a number of different ingredients mostly derived from the plants and some from non vegetable sources. This was an important aspect in the teaching and tanning of all aspiring medical practitioners. Being a great centre of medical teaching Taxila was also well known for a huge variety of medicinal plants growing

---

[145] Said HM. *Al-Beruni's book on pharmacy and Materia Medica. Introduction, commentary and evaluation,* Karachi: Hamdard National Foundation, 1973. p. 38.

in its surroundings. Their recognition, collecting and preparation of medical preparations from herbal sources was an essential part of medical training. The hills surrounding Taxila were where all kind of medicinal vegetable was grown naturally were convenient grounds for collecting useful plants. During the training of doctors careful attention was paid at accurately recognising, gathering, and combining the prescriptions in right proportion. Further emphasis was placed on the proper handling the storage of the raw and prepared medicines. Although there are minerals in Ayurvedic medicines, the vegetable contents utilised are far greater in numbers. Even today the size of the industry dealing with medicines from vegetable and other sources is huge.

The major Sanskrit medical texts have listed over a thousand healing products derived from the plants only. These texts also emphasise how important it is to collect the right constituents from the plants during a particular season and store them properly before using them whenever a prescription has to be prepared. After preparations the medicines were carefully stored and eventually handed over to the patients who needed them. As an example the *Susruta Samhita* has given complex details of preparing an expensive medicine for the eyes, advising its storage in the following words.[146]

> The compound thus prepared is a very good *Anjana* (medicated collyrium) and should be kept in a pure vessel made of ivory, crystal, *Vaidurya, Samkha* (conch shell), stone, gold or silver or Asana wood.

In summary in ancient Ayurvedic medical practice the reach and scope of pharmacy not only required comprehensive knowledge of medicinal agents but their preparations, storage and then careful dispensing to the consumers or patients was of great importance. This in turn

---

[146] See note 120 above, vol. III, p. 99.

had a strong bearing on acquisition and management of an assortment of tools to produce the ultimate produc for the satisfaction of both doctors and their patients. The *Bower Manuscript* described the method of preparing various medicines, where as there is a mention of a wooden pastel as well. When such tools are identified from an archaeological excavation; the site is bound to carry medical significance.

It has been mentioned in previous pages that in Taxila teaching of medicine during a long period of history was well established, where important excavated surgical instruments have also been identified offering a tangible support to its medical standing. At such a site we must also expect that pharmaceutical objects should also surface during excavations. This is not a far fetched assertion and the fact is that a large number of items are in the museum that must have served an obvious pharmaceutical function. A selection of these is discussed below.

Mortar and Pastel

A mortar and pastel is timeless essential house hold equipment used for grinding and pounding herbs and spices, at the same time its use in the preparation of medicines is as old as the use of herbs in the cure of illness. The prescriptions were usually made from a number of vegetable or other organic and non organic materials; these constituents were made into homogeneous palatable powders, pills and potions by crushing in such a device. Its importance is acknowledged to the extent that a mortar and pastel has become an icon that represents a pharmacy. Another interesting aspect is that all over the World this essential apparatus has been evolved in identical looking designs or models by different people to perform same kind of function.

In Taxila a number of pastels and mortars were discovered from pre-Alexandrian site of Bhir Mound and the Greek city of Sirkap, made of hard stone, being indestructible they belonged to extreme of ages. The mortars were from 15 cm to over 25 cm in diameter while there were also numerous pastels of different sizes. Many stone slabs were also found, which must be used for grinding probably spices or similar other materials for domestic uses. There is an unusual saddle shaped grinding slab of stone on display, approximately 40 cm long and 15 cm wide, this might have been used for some special purpose (Fig. 36).

For the pharmaceutical industry an instrument like Mortar and Pastel must be an essential tool and probably this was the reason that quite few such items were found during excavations that may be seen displayed in the museum. Moreover the *Mahavagga* tells us that Buddha himself had specifically given his approval for the use of Mortar and Pastel to his followers. This approval is sufficient to place the simple stone device in a sanctified position in the monasteries.

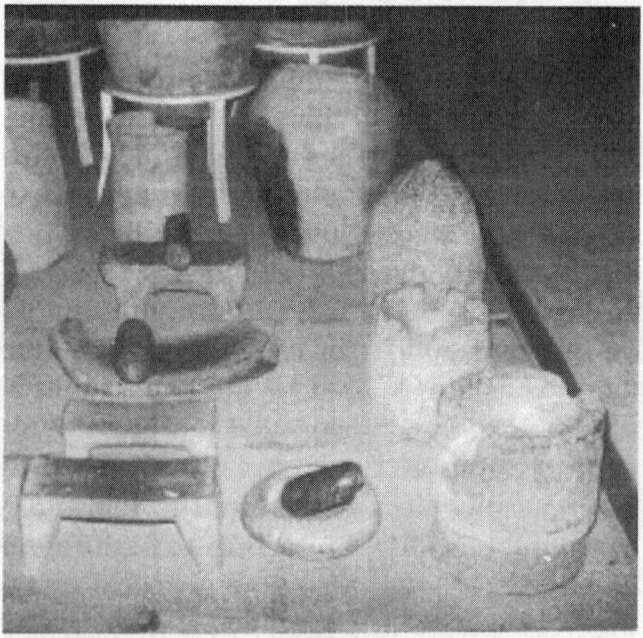

Fig. 36

A mortar and pastel and a saddle shaped grinding stone along with other exhibits in the Taxila Museum

Condensers

There are three condensers of various sizes, one is almost complete and it has been exhibited assembled roughly in the way it must have been used in real life (Fig. 37). It is made of five different components and all may not belong to the same single object rather survived from a number of these devices. The discovery of these devices in large numbers also shows that these were widely used. They are made typically from red clay in the style of other Gandhara pots. The assembled condenser on display stands to a height of about 40 cms. This substantial apparatus, which is unique and cannot be mistaken regarding its function, offers us some understanding of the level of skill of the Gandharan scientists who used it for whatever substance they wanted to purify by the method of evaporation and then condensation. The real intensions are matter of speculation to those who can see this apparatus today. If the Gandharan used it to produce any therapeutic agents or wine, then their achievements are surprisingly exceptional.

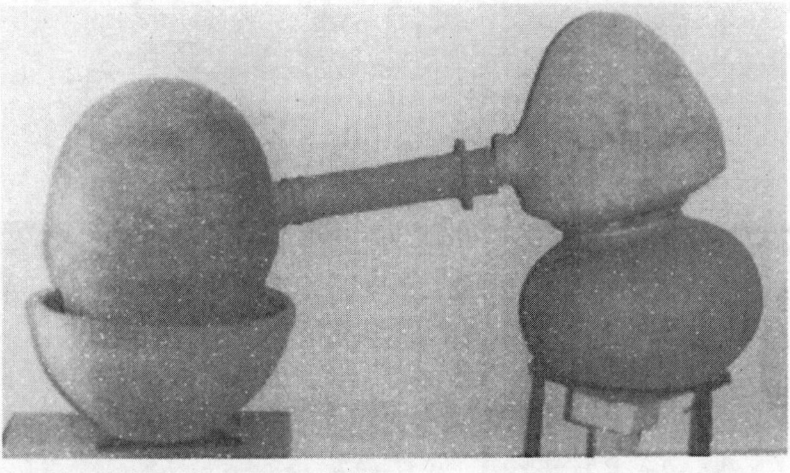

Fig. 37
Condenser made of red clay excavated in Taxila

On another shelf a glass vessel is displayed which looks like a modern condenser similar to those used in chemistry laboratory, with bulging belly, a narrow neck bent at an angle and lipped mouth (Fig. 38). This unusual and mysterious glass vessel is a puzzling exhibit that survived and was excavated in Taxila. It is no doubt a surprising find for the archaeologists because it does not look like other glass vessels and flasks of first or second century CE. The glass manufacturing was not known any where in Gandhara or even any where else in India, where only glass beads or bangles and similar minor glass objects were made. Glass vessels were luxury items that were imported from Roman Empire.[147] The object shown in the picture is also a later find because it is not listed in the catalogue where only a limited number of glass items are listed and illustrated. It might be an interesting pharmaceutical object which justifies further investigation. Its function as a pharmaceutical accessory remains controversial while its mere survival is enigmatic.

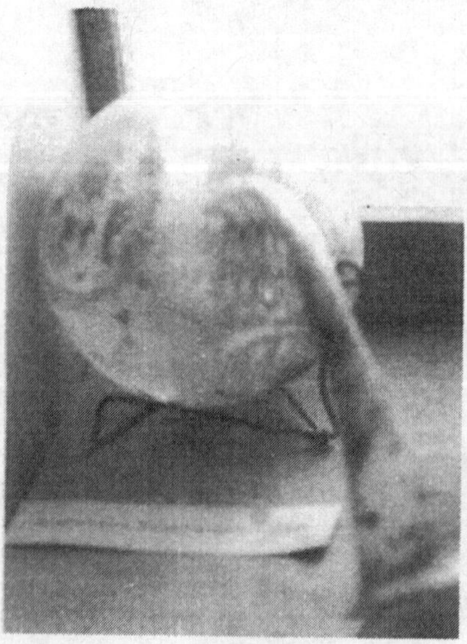

Fig. 38
A glass condenser exhibited in Taxila museum

[147] See note 33 above, vol. II, p. 685.

Storage Jars and other pottery objects

Unlike the rare vessels of glass described previously the pottery jars and other related items of incredible variety in shapes and sizes were discovered in abundance. The tradition of pottery making in the subcontinent goes back to even before the Harappa civilisation. It is now confirmed by the archaeologists who have discovered at Mehrgarh pottery belonging to the Neolithic civilisation in Balochistan.[148] In other words the tradition of pottery making that came down to Gandhara was an old tradition.

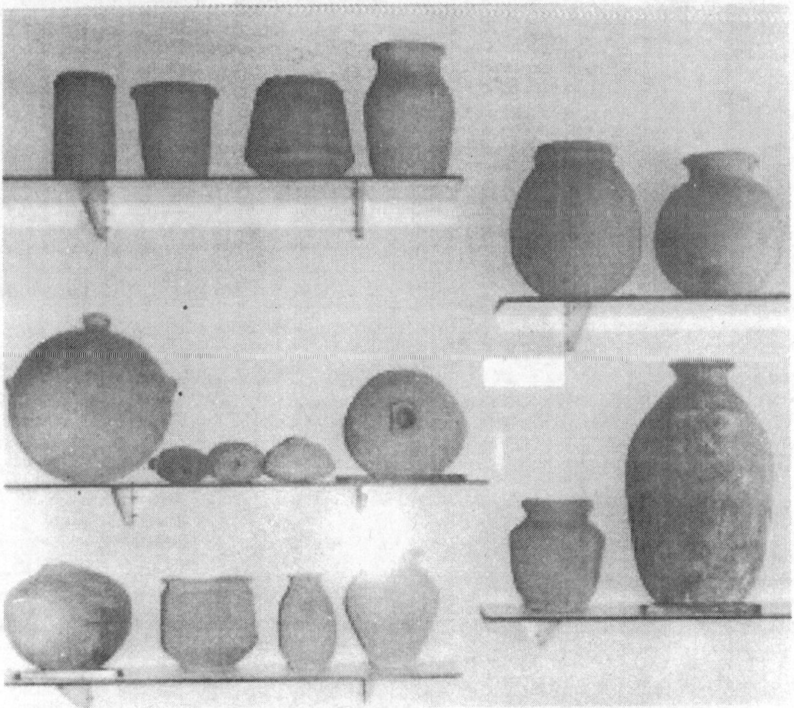

Fig. 39
More storage jars and other pottery objects

All pottery where ever it was discovered in Gandhara has one feature in common, it was made primarily for utility purpose and very little efforts were wasted to enhance it

[148] Kenoyer JM, Heuston K. *The ancient South Asian World*, New York: Oxford University Press, 2005, p.176.

artistically or decorate with motifs. This feature is well demonstrated in Taxila pottery. It was locally made mostly of red clay with much higher sand content.

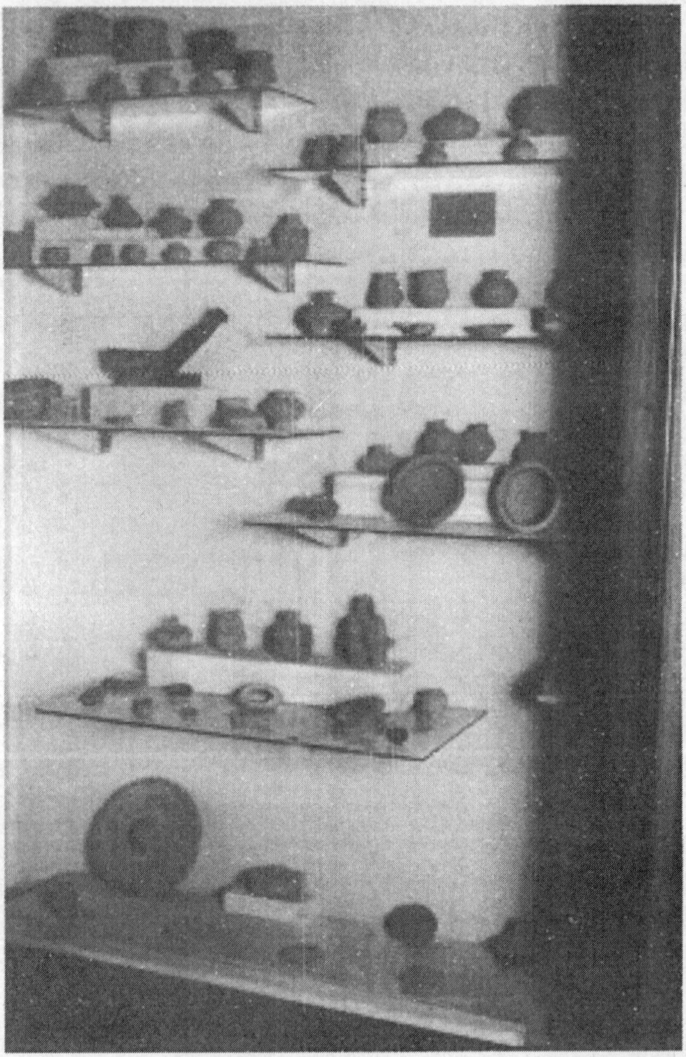

Fig. 40
Some more pottery containers

The accompanied two pictures (Fig. 39 and Fig. 40) give a good indication of the variety in shapes and sizes of pottery vessels that were excavated and exhibited in the museum. Although in two pictures only two displays are represented, there are many other showcases where pottery is displayed. After the stone objects which are probably in largest numbers, the pottery items must be next in their overwhelming presence.

A clay pot in Harappa was discovered, which still contained leaves of a tree that is commonly used for its medicinal properties even today.[149] Such finds offer inimitable evidence that many of the pottery vessels must have been used for storing medicines, a predictable observation. The ultimate evidence of storing medicines in special clay containers was recorded by Sir John Marshall, who discovered an unknown substance in an excavated pot and on analysis it was found to be *salajit,* which even today is peddled by the street quacks as an aphrodisiac.[150] A study of ancient medical texts also tells us that multitudes of medical preparations like pills, powders, potions were used for a variety of therapeutic purposes; it is inevitable that there must be some kind of system in place to store them and transport them. Medicated oil or an unguent can only be handed over to a patient or his (her) close relative in a suitable container. At least some of the hundreds of pottery jars and vessels of all sizes and shapes displayed behind the glass in Taxila Museum must contained some kind of medicine at some time or other. A sensitive chemical analysis from inside these vessels might give valuable insight what once was held in these in the past. The archaeologists have identified some of the pots as oil and wine vessels while some wide mouthed vessels have been described to store unguents. As noted above we learn from the *Bower Manuscript* and other texts that a great many constituents were used to make prescriptions and also about the methods of preparing them. Even a cursory glance into those prescriptions listed in the

---

[149] Chowdhury KA, Ghosh SS. 'Plant remains from Harappa', *Ancient India,* 1947; 7: pp. 3-19.

[150] Marshall, Sir John. *Mohenjo-Daro and the Indus Civilisation,* London: Probsthain, 1931.

texts discussed above may give some idea of the level of the logistics of storing all this material. It will require a vast range of containers first of all to store the medicinal constituents once collected from the plants and mineral or animal origin. Then prepare the prescriptions and finally dispense to the patients the end products in the form of pills, powders or many other assortment of medicines or therapeutic agents that have been repeatedly mentioned.

Taxila is also recognised as a famous centre for the cultivation of medicines of medicinal herbs.[151] These further offer an evidence that some kind of industry for growing and producing medical products existed that obviously will require many kinds of clay pots similar to those in the above pictures and many more can be witnessed displayed in the museum.

Weighing pans and weights

The archaeological evidence clearly shows that the measurement of mass by weighing and that of length by linear measurement were known to the earliest primitive societies. The tools employed by the primeval people in the form of a unit of measurement were their own body parts. The human finger, hand and arm to measure lengths and a small amount held between fingers or handful to measure mass. As the complexity of bartering and trade of goods increased the units of measurements also developed into increasing sophistication. The direct and indirect archaeological evidence confirms that distinct systems of weights and linear measurements existed among most early civilisations such as Egypt, Mesopotamia and that of Indus Valley. The Old Testament provides many references and examples where weights and measure for all kind of domestic uses and commercial purposes were employed. Most ancient religious texts explicitly give emphasis to honesty in weighing when trading with each other.

---

[151] See note 22 above, p. 6.

The excavations of Indus Valley Civilizations have unearthed many stone weights, majority are in the shape of a cube. The abundance of these has helped to clearly understand the system of weights used during the pre-Aryan society. The critical studies of these weights indicate a highly sophisticated system of measuring and weighing was evolved about 5000 years ago. As an example the bricks discovered were uniformly made in a ratio of 4 : 2 : 1, same ratio is also used by the modern brick making industry. The smallest unit of linear measurement ever discovered was also found in Harappa on a scale that on the metric system measures about 1.7 mm.

The huge numbers of cube shaped weights that have been excavated in Harappa and Mohenjodaro and other places were found to be based on a binary system starting from a unit of 0.05, which doubles till reaches 500.[152] But the larger weights were found to be in decimal system.

In archaeological excavations of later periods the discovery of standardised weights made of stone or metals in a variety of shapes is a recurring feature, some of these were found with proper inscription as well.[153] A complete set of weights made of stone and shaped in spherical balls that was discovered in a shop of a jeweller, is also exhibited in the Taxila Museum.

If we examine the weights that have been excavated at various sites right from Mauryan period onwards, we have to acknowledge the fact that the system which was devised by the traders of Indus Valley Civilisation was the fundamental system on which all other were based and with little variations it survived even up to the modern times. Despite many foreign invasions no alien system could replace it until the

---

[152] Kenoyer JM, *Ancient cities of the Indus valley civilization,* American Institute of Pakistan Studies, Oxford: Oxford University Press, 1998. pp. 98-100.

[153] Allchin FR. 'An inscribed weight from Mathura.' *Journal of the Economic and Social History of Orient,* 1964; vol 7: No. 2, pp. 201-5.

metric system that was implemented universally about the middle of the 20th century.

During the pre-Mauryan period two related systems, both having roots from the Indus Valley Civilization were in use. One in the old domain of Kalinga and the other was popular in the kingdom of Magadha. It is recorded by reliable historians that during the Mauryan period standardised weights and measures were adopted by Royal proclamation, these were based on the system that was in use in Kalinga. Exact nature or relationship among these two systems is a matter of historical speculation but these two systems overlapped giving rise to a mixed system that with slight modifications remained in use till modern times. In the back drop of the historical upheavals, multitudes of independent kingdoms, which were continuously in a state of warfare with each other; a uniform system must be in the realm of impossibility. On the other hand trade has to continue despite the chaotic relationship among the states, so the business community must have evolved some practical solutions. This most probably is the reason that same or similar weights and measures used for centuries have been known by names that have discernible similarities.

The ancient medical texts like *Caraka Samhita* or *Susruta Samhita* and the later texts such as the *Astangasangraha,* all have used in their pharmacopoeias weights for solid medical substances and other measures for those medicines that were in liquid form. The *Caraka Samhita* has mentioned two kinds of systems for weights, one from Magadha and the other from Kalinga and has described the system from Magadha to be superior.[154] But in the other two texts there is no differentiation of two systems and most of the names of weights are shared. The reality seems to be that the systems of weights and measures depicted in the extant editions were in fact from the period when the final revisions of these

---

[154] Editorial Board. *The Caraka Samhita,* vol. 5, Jamnagar: Shree Gulabkuverba Ayurvedic Society, 1949, pp. 965-66.

texts were carried out. The last known commentator of the *Caraka Samhita* was Chakrapanidatta, who lived around 1066 CE. While the last reviewer of *Susruta Samhita* was Dalhana, he lived during the 12th century. The last person who completely revised the *Astangasangraha* in about 1220 CE was Arundatta. They existed so close to each other that it must be the reason the present three main Samhitas, *Caraka Samhita, Susruta Samhita* and *Astangasangraha* have common names of the weights and measures. It leaves the *Bower Manuscript* which comes to us in its original form without being revised. In this respect the *Bower Manuscript* must be considered to be older than others because it offers glimpses of the methods of measuring the medicines, perhaps the authors of the *Bower Manuscript* may have borrowed these from the ancient editions of the first two texts mentioned above before they were almost completely revised. A comparison of the weights mentioned in the above medical texts and those objects excavated by the archaeologists would be a useful exercise to understand how the Apothecary of Gandhara weighed the medical constituents and prepared the prescription. The above texts with the exception of the *Bower Manuscript* begin their systems of weights from an imaginative and impractical concept of a single speck of dust which, increases in numbers or weight in ratios of 8, 6, 4, and 2 but not in a consistent sequence. It is demonstrated in following systems.

The *Caraka Samhita* has elaborated a system of weights that starts from a particle of dust or *Vamsi* progressing as illustrated below.

6 *Vamsi* or *Dhvamsi*	=	1 *Marici*
6 *Marici*	=	1 rape seed or Sarsapa
8 rape seeds	=	1 grain of rice
2 rice grains	=	1 black gram grain
2 black gram	=	1 barley seed or yava
4 barley seeds	=	1 Andika

4 *Andika*	=	1 *Masaka* or *Dhanyaka* or *Masha*
4 *Masaka*	=	1 *Sana*
2 *Sana*	=	1 *Dranksana* or *Kola* or *Badara*
2 *Dranksana*	=	1 *Karsa* or *Aksa* or *Tinduka*
2 *Karsa*	=	1 *Sukti*
2 *Sukti*	=	1 *Pala* or *Musti*
2 *Pala*	=	1 *Prasrta*
2 *Prasrta*	=	1 *Anjali* or *Kudava*
4 *Anjali*	=	1 *Prastha*
4 *Prastha*	=	1 *Adhaka* or *Patra*
2 *Adhaka*	=	1 *Kasana*
4 *Kasdana*	=	I *Drona* or *Ghata*
2 *Drona*	=	1 *Surpa* or *Kumbha*
2 *Surpa*	=	1 *Goni* or *Khari* or *Vaha*

The *Susruta Samhita* does not elaborates on any particular system of weights similar to *Caraka Samhita* as listed above or an increasing values of weights from a conceptual dust particle, but has mentioned following weights whenever the constituents of prescriptions are to be mixed together. These weights that are used in *Susruta Samhita* are common with the system of *Caraka Samhita* and there is no differentiation of two different systems as pointed out by some of the authors. The following weights for solid substances are often mentioned in *Susruta Samhita.*

Masha
Aksha or *Aksa*
Sukti
Pala
Kudava or *Anjali*

The *Susruta Samhita* contains many examples of prescriptions where the weights of ingredients are recorded before these are mixed according to the required amounts. The forthcoming example illustrates the general trend and not much dissimilar to what is contained in the other texts cited above.[155]

> A *Prastha* measure of oil duly prepared by cooking it with half a *Kudava* measure of *yava* (barley), half a *Pala* weight of mangishtha and a 100 *Prastha* measure of amla.

The modern English translation of *Astangasangraha* has used the systems of weights almost same as listed by *Caraka Samhita* only with minor alteration. The translator has also tagged a table of weights in the appendix.[156] This table shows many of the weights converted into metric system as well, although the conversions do not appear to be very accurate, because there are obvious wide variations which seem to be far beyond the threshold of mathematical tolerance.

The sketchy approach to the weights by which the medicines are measured mentioned by the multiple authors of the *Bower Manuscript* is represented by the limited number of weights that have been recorded when preparing the prescriptions; a fact may be witnessed all the way through the text. It seems that absolute accuracy by actually weighing the ingredients was not intended. Moreover the unworkable extremely small weights like a grain of sand or larger weights on the opposite side of the scale are altogether ignored, utilising only those that fall in the middle of the scale and utilised in day to day use. Such matter-of-fact approach has been employed throughout the pharmacopoeia of the *Bower Manuscript*.

As an example the first weight on the scale described is *Karsha* or *Karsa*, is equal to quarter of a *Pala* and has been

---

[155] See note 120 above.

[156] *Astangasamgraha of Vagbhata*, vol. III, Murthy KRS. tr., Varanasi: Chowkhamba Orientalia, 19??, Appendix 12.

derived from the expression of 'cat paw' or a little of something. While *Pala* which is probably the most commonly used measurement for medicines is also known as *Mushti,* a handful or a fistful. Likewise the names of few other weights also appear to be from a primary Sanskrit root representing various positions of human hand. The measurement of substances using hand and fingers seem to be used often. A prescription from the *Bower Manuscript* quoted below offers a good example how the chosen constituents were measured and then mix together to produce a final therapeutic product. We must not be concerned as regard to the merits of the formula and the number of medical conditions it is supposed to cure without any recommendation of its dose; it is only quoted to demonstrate the typical method of weighing as much as a dozen ingredients to make a final salutary formula of a curative remedy.[157]

> The *Shadva* powder, take a *Karsha* each of tamarind, dry ginger, Indian sorrel, pomegranate and sour jujube, one half *Karsha* coriander seed, sonchal salt, cumin seed and cinnamon, one hundred *Pala* of black pepper, powder them together with four *Pala* of sugar. This powder cleans the tongue. It is a cordial and promotes the appetite. It also cures severe pain in the heart, spleen and sides and removes retention of discharges, relives cough and asthma and being astringent stops chronic diarrhoea and haemorrhoids.

It is just one example selected from the *Bower Manuscript* where ingredients are weighed before they are mixed together in similar fashion.

It is evident that the tradition of weighing the medicines must be a standard practice in Gandhara where the *Bower Manuscript* was compiled. The archaeological finds in Taxila of fairly small balance pans and corresponding smaller weights, offers further corroborated verification that small enough weighing pans and corresponding weights suitable for weighing medicines were in common use.

[157] See note 49 above, p.78.

Many weighing pans were discovered that are recorded in the catalogue and can also be seen displayed in the museum. These are all for hanging from a vertical beam which was probably wooden, because metal vertical beam for a balance have not been excavated. Three of such weighing pans are of interest because these due to their sizes might be used for weighing medicines. These are 2, 5 cm, 5 cm and 6 cm in diameter. These small pans are badly damaged owing to the thin metal plate of copper they were made. In contrast all the weights that have been excavated in Gandhara and particularly in Taxila were customarily made of granite, chert or similar harder type of stone that was available locally. Another peculiarity of the stone weights from Gandhara excavations is that they are all spherical in shape, while the weights from Indus Valley Civilisation were always cubical and most weights discovered out side Gandhara were conical shaped. The experts have not come up any logical explanation as to why an absolute spherical shape of the weights was chosen by the designers of weights in Gandhara. The rounded ball-like weights also exhibit a round hole that in many instances was found to have lead fillings to adjust for corrections. This feature is common in the ancient and modern weights and confirms that even in the distant past strict inspection was in place to make sure the weights used by the trades were accurate.

The number of weights discovered during the Taxila excavations is more than found in any other site of comparable period. The numbers are enough to study the relationship of the ratios and decisively determine the system of the weights. Moreover 25 weights were also fond in a place that was recognised as a jeweller's shop. From these a complete set of weights has been constructed which, illustrates that the smaller weights suitable to measure precious materials in a jeweller's shop or even medicines follow a binary sequence or the next weight is a product of previous weight multiplied by two. The smallest weights are averaged to the value of 3.1 gram in metric system. This is also the median weight of basic silver coins excavated at a number of sites and was standardised during the time of Mauryan Empire. From this smallest there is sequential increase in the ratio of 1, 2, 4, 8, 16, 32, and 64. But the higher weights follow a decimal system where the successive higher weight is the product of multiplication by 10 of its previous number and follow in the ratio of 160, 320, 640 or 1600, 3200, 6400 etc. A close study of the system of weights excavated from Taxila brings about an interesting truth that the basic system of weights remained the same which was devised more than 5000 years ago during the Indus Valley Civilisation.

Once more the textual evidence contained in the above mentioned medical manuscripts seem to be fully corroborated with the actual weights and the tiny pans discovered during the archaeological excavations. There can be little doubt that the weights at smaller or lower echelon also match the tiny sizes of the balance pans that may be seen among the exhibits. The smaller weights and pans must have been used for weighing the medicines or other precious substances.

All the medical compendiums have mentioned with little variation most of the weights that have been discussed above. The discovery of corresponding weights at numerous archaeological sites in Gandhara is a clear indication that the physicians of Gandhara were careful to weigh and measure the medicines before these were prepared and finally administered to the patients.

It is intriguing how information from the ancient texts when studied in the light of the archaeological finds would complement each other and can lead to discover interesting realities and interpretations of the past.

Appendix
Surgical Instrument in the Taxila Museum

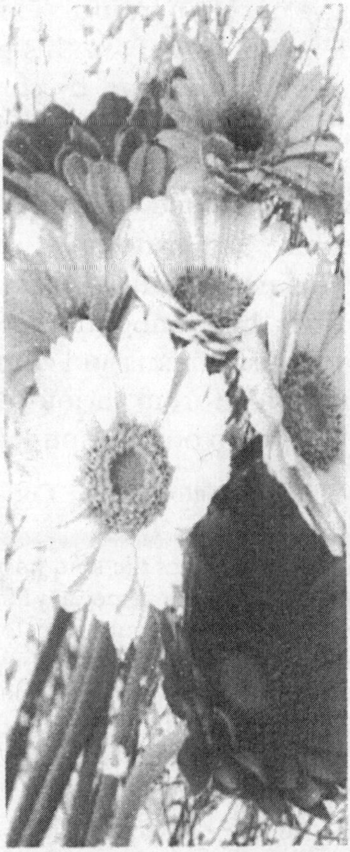

There is substantial historical evidence to support the prevalence of surgical practice during ancient times in the subcontinent of India. However, in contrast to the contemporaneous Greek and Roman periods, there is a notable absence of any archaeological finds in the form of surgical instruments. Inquiries to major museums and personal contacts have not been fruitful. This lack of relevant archaeological evidence of surgery in this part of the world is surprising. It cannot be explaind by climatic conditions alone, since museums are full of metal objects that were excavated in a reasonably preserved state. Girindranath Mukhopadhyaya has commented, "as far as I have been able to trace, our museums contain no finds supplying us with any information".[1] Acknowledging a complete absence of any archaeological finds, his monograph relies on numerous illustrations of surgical instruments and compares these with modern instruments copied from various catalogues of the period. This paper reports on one exceptional archaeological

* Dr. Nasim H Naqvi, FRCA, Heaton Grange Cottage, Heaton Grange Drive, Bolton, BL 15DA; UK.

The author gratefully acknowledges the kind hospitality and untiring help from the staff of the Taxila Museum, especially Mr Abdul Ghafoor and Dr. Mohammad Ashraf Khan, PhD, Deputy Director, Archaeology and Museums, Government of Pakistan, for permission to photograph the exhibits. The valuable professional help during the photography provided by Khalil A Khana of Islamabad is gratefully acknowledged. My thanks also to A Humphries, of the Thackray Medical Museum, Leeds, who supplied the pictures of modern decapitating hooks.

[1] G Mukhopadhyaya. 'The surgical instruments of the Hindus with a comparative study of the surgical instruments of the Greek' in JB Khanna, ed., *Roman, Arab, and the modern European surgeons,* New Delhi: RK Nahar, 1977, p. iv.

site where surgical instruments and other medical equipment have been discovered; it was also a known seat of medical education.

Taxila is one of the most important archaeological sites in the subcontinent. It is situated about 20 km north of Pakisan's capital, Islamabad. The original archaeological survey and excavations were carried out before the Second World War by Sir John Marshall (1876-1958), who meticulously recorded the discoveries and historical details in three volumes.[2] The excavations continue, yet even such prolonged activity has not uncovered all that is still hidden under the earth. The archaeological sits comprise three main townships and many smaller ruins, scattered in a radius of about 10 km. The earliest site is Bhir Mound, which, as revealed by recent excavations, was built on a Stone Age settlement. The second is a Greek town called Sirkap, and the third only partially excavated site is a Kushan settlement called Sirsukh.

Taxila gained importance and prosperity because of its strategic position on the main trade routes. It is mentioned in the ancient texts with its original name Taksasila.[3] The Greeks gave it the present name of Taxila. When Cyrus expanded his empire, around 560 BC, Taxila came under Persian control. Herodotus tells us that it was the twentieth and richest province in the empire of Darius I.[4] In 326 BC Alexander came to Taxila, received a lavish welcome, and stayed to rest and replenish supplies for is army. Within a decade of his death, Taxila was under the Mauryan dynasty, and Asoka made it a great centre of Buddhism, which was

---

[2] J Marshall. *Taxila: an illustrated account of archaeological excavations,* (3 volumes), Cambridge University Press, 1951. See vol. 2, pp. 570, 577, 595, 599 and 601,

[3] H Raychaudhuri. *Political history of ancient India,* Delhi: Oxford University Press, 1996, pp. 54-9.

[4] Herodotus. *The history,* D Grene, University of Chicago Press, 1987, Book 3, p. 94.

exported to China and beyond. After the decline of Mauryan power. Taxila remained under the Bactrian Greeks, Parthians, Sakas and Kushans, respectively for more than 400 years. According to legend, the Apostle Thomas brought his mission to the court of Gondophares, king of Taxila.[5] In the early fifth century AD, Taxila was sacked, burnt and thoroughly destroyed by the Huns, probably the descendants of Hsiungnu people from Central Asia. Earthquakes caused further extensive physical damage that buried the city until its discovery in the late nineteenth century.

Some Buddhist sacred books have described Taxila as a place of learning or a university town.[6] Its standing as a centre of excellence for medical education is well documented.[7] Among the legendary medical personages associated with Taxila, Atreya and his pupil Jivaka are frequently mentioned in ancient medical literature.[8] A number of Jatakas pay homage to Jivaka, who rose to become physician to the Buddha.[9] Another renowned figure is Caraka, who is best known as the complier of *Caraka Samhita*.[10] According to modern medical historians, the *Caraka Samhita* tradition has been associated with Taxila.[11] Caraka flourished during the reign of Kanishka, who ruled from 100 to 126 AD, and is also known to have laid the foundations of Sirsukh, the third

[5] JN Farquhar. 'The Apostle Thomas in North India', *John Rylands Library Bulletin,* 1926, pp. 80-111.

[6] H Oldenberg *Sacred books of the east: The Mahavagga,* T W Rhys Davids, Tr., Oxford Clarendon Press, 1882, pp. 184-7.

[7] RK Mookerji. *Ancient Indian education,* London: Macmillan, 1947, pp. 468-78.

[8] G J Meulenbeld. *History of Indian medical literature,* (3 volumes), Groningen Egbert Forsten, 1999, vol. 1A, pp. 126-7, 693.

[9] V Fausboll. *The Jataka: together with its commentary, being tales of anterior births of Gotama Buddha,* (7 volumes), T W Rhys Davids, tr., London: Trubner, 1877-97, p. 175.

[10] See note 8 above, vol.1 A, pp. 120-3.

[11] R Porter. *The greatest benefit to mankind,* London: Harper Collins, 1997. p. 138.

settlement in Taxila. The discovery of surgical instruments at this ancient seat of medical education offers additional and unequivocal validation of its standing in surgical practice.

All the metal object discovered in Taxila were analysed and the result recorded. The instruments that are the subject of this paper were made of almost pure copper.[12] Copper smelting was known in the region and, according to Marshal, "metallurgical skill had reached a high level."[13] A large number of other copper object were also excavated, which are exhibited in the Taxila Museum. This small museum, rich in the quality of its exhibits, is the only place in the subcontinent where we can see excavated surgical instruments.

Probably the earliest surgical instruments ever discovered belong to the Aegean civilization (1400 BC) and were made of bronze.[14] Many copper-alloy and iron instruments of Greek origin, and much more refined and complex Roman instruments, may be seen in a number of European museums; some of these will be compared with the instruments discovered in Taxila.

In all, thirteen objects are displayed in the Taxila Museum under the heading of surgical instrument, twelve are illustrated in Figure 1. The one not included is the fragment of a handle of some unknown object. Another of the exhibits (Figure 1: C) is not a surgical instrument, but a device used during offerings to the gods.[15] An account of the remaining eleven instruments follows.

---

[12] See note 2 above, vol. 2, p. 577.

[13] See note 2 above, vol. 2, p. 570.

[14] R Arnott. 'Surgical practice in the prehistoric Aegean', *Medizinhist J.*, 1997, 32: 249-78.

[15] See note 2 above, vol. 2, p. 595.

Decapitators

A "decapitator" is a modern term, introduced by British authors during the nineteenth century; their descriptions of and modifications to this instrument are fully documented.[16] On the other hand, Europeans described a similar device used in the same circumstances with its ancient name, a hook knife, embryo hook or *Scharfer Haken* (sharp hook).[17] This instrument was designed to cut through the neck of the dead foetus during severely obstructed labour. A further modification of this device is a saw-tooth edge at the inner border.

The decapitators excavated in Taxila are the most important, unique and interesting instruments in the collection. Their use as such is highly plausible, despite Sir John Marshall's own archaeological evaluation of these objects: "The purpose of these curious-looking instruments is by no means certain, but the accepted view, which the writer does not share, is that they were surgical decapitators for use in obstetric operations".[18]

Six such instruments were excavated and are listed in Marshall's catalogue; three are not on display. Two of these were discovered as fragments, approximately 5.5 cm in length, and made of copper sheeting strengthened with copper-wire rib. These fragments were found at the oldest site of Bhir Mound and were dated to the third to second century BC. This means that such a device was in use before the invasion of Alexander. The third was excavated complete, measuring 17.5 cm in length, and made of solid copper with a round handle ending in a disc. It was discovered at the Sirkap site and pertains to the first century

[16] B Hibbard. *The obstetrician's armamentarium,* San Anselmo, CA: Norman Publishing, 2000, pp. 254-9.

[17] W Kuhn, U Trohler. eds., *Armamentarium obstetricium Gottingense,* Gottingen: Vandenhoek and Ruprecht, 1987, p. 119.

[18] See note 2 above, vol. 2, pp. 599-601.

AD. This and one of the fragments described above are illustrated in the catalogue.

Of the other three in the display, two lack handles (Figure 1: K and L), although both are shown in Marshall's account with handles, which must have been lost at some later stage. Including the handles, their length was recorded as 16.5 cm, without them, they measure about 6 cm and 7.5 cm respectively. They were discovered at two different sites in Sirkap. Both of these blades appear to be distorted, presumbly due to ageing and metal stress. One clearly shows a crack at the outer edge in the line of strees (Figure 1: K) and was dated to the early first century BC; the other slightly bigger one was found in layers of the first or second century AD (Figure 1: L).

The sixth decapitator is almost complete and is robustly constructed instrument of solid copper (Figure 1: D, and 2). It was discovered in the second stratum at Sirkap, dating to the first century AD. This distinctive instrument is 16.5 cm long, with a strong round handle, terminating in a disc; its curved blade is sharp inside and blunt outside. The blade shows considerable damage and loss at the end (Figure 3), it also differs slightly in shape from the two fragments discussed above. The handles of all such instruments, irrespective of their period, have some unique common features; they are made of solid copper, uniform in length, round in cross section and terminate in a disc.

There is abundant historical evidence to support the use of a sharp embryo hook knife or decapitator in specific circumstances. The following statement is found in the Susruta Samhita, where a full chapter is devoted to the management of obstructed labour and surgical removal of the dead foetus.

An intelligent physician should not waste a single moment in drawing out the foetus, as soon as it would be found to be dead in the womb, since neglect in such cases leads to the instantaneous death of the mother, like an animal dying of suffocation. An erudite physician, well versed in anatomy, should use in such cases a mandalagra instrument for the purpose of cutting out (the foetus), since a sharp-edged vrddhi-patra may some times hurt the mother during the operation.[19]

The "mandalagra" has been described as a decapitator by a later author.[20] Caraka mentioned an operative procedure for extracting the dead foetus, in the chapter *Sarirasthana* of the *Caraka Samhita,* but without naming a special instrument.[21]

In his book *De medicine,* the Roman medical writer, Aulus Cornelious Celsus (early to mid first century AD), described a sharp hook knife and the use of such an instrument to sever the neck of the dead foetus:

> The remedy then is to cut through the neck, in order that the two parts may be extracted separately. This is done with a hook, which resembles the one mentiond above, but has all its inner edge sharp. Then we must proceed to extract the head first, then the rest.[22]

Soranus of Ephesus (AD 98-138), the earliest writer on obstetrics and gynaecology, recommended embryotomy and the use of hooks to extract the dead foetus.[23] Paul of Aegineta (seventh century AD), who followed Aetius of Amida (sixth century AD), also recommended embryotomy

---

[19] KK Bhishagratna. ed. and tr., *Susruta Samhita,* (3 volumes), Varanasi, Chaukhamba Sanskrit Series Office, 1981, vol. 2, p. 407. ch. 15, verse 16.

[20] K Das. *Obstetric forceps: its history and evolution,* Leeds: Medical Museum, 1993 (first published in 1929), p. 9. See also note 1 above, p. 174.

[21] AC Kaviratna, P Sharma. eds. and trs., *Caraka Samhita,* Delhi: Sri Satguru Publications, 1996, p. 524; ch. 8, verse 31.

[22] WG Spencer. ed. and tr., *Celsus De medicina,* London: William Heinemann, 1938, pp. 459-60.

[23] O Temkin. tr., *Sranus' Gynecology,* Baltimore: Johns Hopkins University Press, 1956, pp. 189-96.

in a similar situation, without mentioning a special instrument.[24] During the tenth century AD, Albucasis gave details of a hook and a variety of special knives for embryotomy during obstructed labour when foetal death had occurred.[25]

Archaeological evidence of comparable Roman instruments is useful in evaluting those found at Taxila. An embryo hook discovered at Pompeii was first described and illustrated by Vulpes in 1847.[26] Its handle was of copper alloy, its hook of iron, and it was originally 17 cm long; its present length after damage is 7.7 cm. Bliquez lists the same instrument along with five other embryo hooks in his catalogue of Roman surgical instruments.[27] All are exhibited at the National Archaeological Museum of Naples. Unfortunately only their handles have survived and none retains the hook. These Roman instruments are all blunt type embryo hooks and it seems that no sharp embryo hook of Roman origin as described by Celsus has ever been identified. A mysterious illustration of a sharp hook is a source of confusion due to the ambiguous account by Milne, "a knife on this principle is in the Bibliotheque Nationale."[28] The legend under the illustration reads, "after Vedrenes". This is a reference to the French translation of *De medicine* by A Vedrenees, published in 1876.[29] The book contains many pictures of Roman instruments from Pompeii,

---

[24] F Adms. tr., *The seven books of Paulus Aegineta,* (3 volumes), London: Sydenham Society, 1844-47, vol. 1, p. 648.

[25] MS Spink, GL Lewis. trs., *Albucasis on surgery and instruments,* London: Wellcome Institute of the History of Medicine, 1973, pp. 492-93.

[26] B Vulpes. *Illustrazione di tutti gli strumenti chirurgici scavati in Erolano e in Pompei,* Napoli: Stamperia Reale, 1847, p. 81.

[27] LJ Bliquez. *Roman surgical instruments and other minor objects in the National Archaeological Museum of Naples,* Mainz: Verlag Philipp von Zabern, 1994, pp. 129-30.

[28] JS Milne. *Surgical instruments in Greek and Roman times,* Oxford: Clarendon Press, 1907, p. 154.

[29] A Vedrenes. tr., *Traite de medecine de A.C. Celse,* Paris: G Masson, 1876.

including the embryo hook Vulpes listed, but no sharp hook similar to Milne's illustration is depicted anywhere.

The German scholar, Ernst Kunzl, has illustrated an instrument from the Byzantine period, in the collection at Jena, labelled *Großer Haken.*[30] It is not a sharp hook, though it appears remarkably similar to the instrument from Taxila.

Some of the references and quotes discussed above clearly suggest that embryotomy was practised in ancient times, and, in desperate circumstances, a hook knife, sharp inside and blunt outside, was employed to facilitate delivery of a dead foetus. The instrument from Taxila appears to fit the description (Figure 2).

Decapitators have been used even in modern obstetrics and were listed in British surgical instrument catalogue until the middle of the twentieth century under the names "Ramsbottom's Decapitating Hook" and "Jardine's Decapitating Hook" (Figure 4).[31] These modern 30 cm long instruments were sharp inside, blunt outside, and strongly made. It is astonishing that this device remains virtually unchanged, and has been used and repeatedly mentioned by surgeons of different civilizations for almost 2000 years.

Probes

Three objects displayed in the Taxila Museum may have a surgical application as probes (Figure 1: H, I and J). Although they show no striking similarities with documented Greek or Roman probes, they still resemble them.[32] Two are finely made and in good condition (Figure 1: I and J), about 9 cm and 7 cm long. The third is thicker and badly

---

[30] E Kunzl. *Medizinische Instrumente aus Sepulkralfunden der romischen Kaiserzeit,* Cologne: Rheinland, 1983, p. 52.

[31] CF Thackray. *Catalogue of surgical instruments and appliances,* Leeds: C F Thackray, 1935, p. 117.

[32] LJ Bliquez. *Roman instruments and minor objects in the university of Mississippi,* Gotenborg: Paul Astroms, 1988, p. 74.

damaged (Figure 1: H), measuring 6.5 cm, and may not have a surgical application. All are made of pure copper and may have had wooden handles. The date and site of excavation of these probes cannot be ascertained as they are not included in Marshall's catalogue and were probably discovered after the original excavations. It has been suggested that the puncturing or lancing of boils is alluded to in the Vedic literature.[33] It is a reasonable assumption that pointed probes were developed later for various surgical uses.

Spatulae

Marshall listed five spatulate under surgical instruments.[34] All bear a decoration of typical Buddhist design at the end of the handle. One illustrated in his catalogue has a heart shaped hole in the blade, the other two are missing. The remaining two in the display are similar (Figure 1: A and B), having flat, oval blades measuring 22 cm and 20 cm respectively. All the spatulae were found at Sirkap, in layers associated with the first or second century AD. In size and shape, items A and B are comparable with Roman spatulae, excavated in large numbers and seen in many museums and collection.[35] However, their use in some religious rites cannot be ruled out.

There are another three objects among the exhibits (Figure 1: E, F and G), these are not listed, dated or described in the catalogue, and must have been discovered during later excavations. Two are similar in shape and size (Figure 1: E and F) about 13.5 cm and 14.5 cm in length, the third (Figure 1: G) has a shorter handle of 9 cm. All three are made of copper, and have rounded blades of equal

---

[33] KG Zysk. *Religious medicine: the history and evolution of Indian medicine*, New Brunswick: Transaction Publishers, 1993, p. 227.

[34] See note 2 above, vol. 2, p. 600.

[35] R Jackson. 'Roman doctors and their instruments: recent research into ancient practice', *J. Roman Archaeology*, 1990, 3: 5-27.

size. Their handles are plain and lack any features or decoration, and are square in cross section, quite unlike those of the decapitators and spatulae. They resemble an 11 cm long instrument, listed by Milne as a tongue depressor.[36] In shape, design and weight they are totally different from many domestics appliances exhibited in the museum and it is difficult to imagine these had any domestic or trade application. One can only speculate that these esoteric objects may have been used as ointment applicators, tongue depressors or retractors.

Among those objects not on display (many are kept in the depository) but included in the catalogue, a few may have a surgical application. A copper forceps about 8 cm long looks similar to Greek or Roman forceps. This is made from a single long strip of copper, which is bent in the middle giving a springy quality, a ring below the loop further strengthens its stability. It was found in stratum II (early first century BC), in the Greek town of Sirkap. The surgical use of this forceps cannot be established with certainty, but it is listed under surgical instruments, while others made of iron are described as tweezers and listed elswhere.

Under the heading "iron objects", the catalogue shows a few badly damaged knives, which might be razors or domestic knives, Razors, however, were used for surgical operations. A French team of archaeologists excavated, among other medical artefacts, a scalpel at a site in Afghanistan contemporary with Taxila during the reign of Kanishka.[37] This object is not similar to a typical Roman surgical knife, but, since it has a blade at one end and an olivary probe at the other, it could have been used in ancient surgery.[38] If it had a surgical application then it is the only

[36] See note 28 above, p. 79.

[37] O Guillaume, A Rougeulle. *Fouilles D' Ai Khanoum,* Paris: De Boccard, 1987, Pl. XI, figure 6.

[38] R Jackspon. Curator of Romano-British collections, British Museum, London, personal communication, Jan. 2002.

scalpel ever discovered outside the Greek and Roman civilizations. Its existence in the same period as some of the instruments discovered in Taxila offers convincing evidence that surgical instruments were designed and manufactured in the region.

Needles for suturing wounds, were used in antiquity.[39] In Taxila needles for domestic use were excavated, but Marshall has catalogued under surgical instruments three needles that were discovered at the earliest township of Bhir Mound in stratum IV belonging to the third or second centuries BC.[40] They are 5 cm to 7 cm in length, and made of copper with a rounded eye.

In addition, there are many implements such as weighing pans, pestles and mortars, medicine jars, condensers, and a peculiar looking pottery object with four spouts, which may be an inhaler. Some of these must have been used to weigh, manufacture, store or dispense pharmacoutical agents. These objects deserve further investigation.

---

[39] TA Wise. *Commentary on the Hindu system of medicine,* Calcutta: The Baptist Mission Press, 1845, p. 171. See also *Susruta Samhita,* Sutrasthana, ch. 8, verses 3-4, on needles.

[40] See note 2 above, vol. 2, p. 601.

INDEX

J

K

L

M

N

O

P

R

S

T